AF803104

A THEORY OF METAPHOR

Truth, Falsity, and the Uncanny

Fredric V. Bogel

Routledge
Taylor & Francis Group
LONDON AND NEW YORK

Designed cover image: cerber82, Getty

First published 2026
by Routledge
4 Park Square, Milton Park, Abingdon, Oxon OX14 4RN

and by Routledge
605 Third Avenue, New York, NY 10158

Routledge is an imprint of the Taylor & Francis Group, an informa business

© 2026 Fredric V. Bogel

The right of Fredric V. Bogel to be identified as author of this work has been asserted in accordance with sections 77 and 78 of the Copyright, Designs and Patents Act 1988.

All rights reserved. No part of this book may be reprinted or reproduced or utilised in any form or by any electronic, mechanical, or other means, now known or hereafter invented, including photocopying and recording, or in any information storage or retrieval system, without permission in writing from the publishers.

Trademark notice: Product or corporate names may be trademarks or registered trademarks, and are used only for identification and explanation without intent to infringe.

British Library Cataloguing-in-Publication Data
A catalogue record for this book is available from the British Library

Library of Congress Cataloging-in-Publication Data

Names: Bogel, Fredric V., 1943- author
Title: A theory of metaphor: truth, falsity, and the uncanny / Fredric V. Bogel.
Description: Abingdon, Oxon; New York: Routledge, 2025. | Includes bibliographical references and index. | Identifiers: LCCN 2025007727 (print) | LCCN 2025007728 (ebook) | ISBN 9781032908403 hardback | ISBN 9781032909004 paperback | ISBN 9781003560050 ebook
Subjects: LCSH: Metaphor | Truthfulness and falsehood | Uncanny, The (Psychoanalysis)
Classification: LCC PN228.M4 B64 2025 (print) | LCC PN228.M4 (ebook)
LC record available at https://lccn.loc.gov/2025007727
LC ebook record available at https://lccn.loc.gov/2025007728

ISBN: 978-1-032-90840-3 (hbk)
ISBN: 978-1-032-90900-4 (pbk)
ISBN: 978-1-003-56005-0 (ebk)

DOI: 10.4324/9781003560050

Typeset in Times New Roman
by Deanta Global Publishing Services, Chennai, India

Tell all the truth but tell it slant—
Success in Circuit lies

Emily Dickinson

CONTENTS

Acknowledgements *ix*

1 Introduction: A Theory of Metaphor 1

2 Processing Metaphor: Resistance and Interpretation 15

3 Metaphor and Biblical Interpretation 27

4 The Persistence of the Tenor: Falsity in Truth 35

5 The Decline of Literal Truth and Reference 42

6 Poems as Metaphors: To Truth through Fiction 47

7 The Double Transit of Metaphor: Metaphor and the Uncanny 54

8 Novelty and the End State of Metaphor: Uncanny Doubling 66

9 The Uncanny: Psychoanalytic and Metaphoric 76

10 Metaphor and Affect: The Uncanny, Paradox, Wonder, Religion 83

11 Conclusion 89

Appendix 95
Bibliography 98
Index 105

ACKNOWLEDGEMENTS

This expression of heartfelt gratitude would doubtless have been longer if I had not written *A Theory of Metaphor* after retiring from the Cornell University English Department to a sea island off the coast of South Carolina. But that relative solitude has made possible stretches of concentrated reading and writing from which full-time teaching and a vibrant university community might have—pleasurably, to be sure—distracted me.

I am grateful to my colleague Kevin Attell for his friendship and intellectual generosity, and particularly for alerting me to the significance of Hans Blumenberg's important work on metaphor; to my friend and former graduate student, Christina Black, for many conversations about literature, criticism, and theory, and in particular for her own writing on metaphor; to my son, Alexander Bogel, who shared an important insight into metaphor and the unconscious at a key early moment; to my wife, Catherine Burroughs, who took time from her own academic and fictional writing to proofread, edit, advise, and—most important—tirelessly discuss innumerable connections among metaphor, typology, psychoanalysis, the uncanny, and more; to Jonathan Culler, for his brilliant writings on metaphor and other modes of figuration, his suggestions about the form of this project, and his friendship and support during many years as colleague and friend; to Michael Ferber, for sharing an early version of his splendid book, *Poetry and Language: The Linguistics of Verse*, with its learned and lucid chapter on metaphor, and for his shrewd comments on a portion of the present study; to Debra Fried, invaluable friend and colleague, exemplar of imaginative close reading, deep student of metaphor and figurative language, and continuous fountain of inventive discussion and warm support; to physical therapist Doug Miller, who boldly led me where I would never have thought to go—to *Star Trek: The Next Generation*; to Karen Raith, Senior Editor at Routledge, for whose enthusiasm, support, and humaneness I will always be deeply grateful; to Chris Ratcliffe, Editorial Assistant at Routledge, whose exactness, promptness, kindness, and professionalism have made our almost daily exchanges both efficient and pleasurable; and to Anna Callander, Production Editor, and Sarah Pearsall, Copy Editor, for their professional care in shaping this book into its final form.

1

INTRODUCTION

A Theory of Metaphor

The responses that metaphor has called forth from readers and writers are nearly as varied as the figure of speech itself. Aristotle views metaphor as an agreeable means to the acquisition of knowledge:

> To learn easily is naturally pleasant to all people, and words signify something, so whatever words create knowledge in us are pleasurable … Metaphor most brings about learning … [It] especially has clarity and sweetness and strangeness.
>
> *(Aristotle on Rhetoric 1405a, 200; 1410b, 218)*

To Robert Frost, metaphor has even seemed to be "all there is of thinking … The richest accumulation of the ages is the noble metaphors we have rolled up" (Frost, "Education by Poetry" 725). In a more aesthetic mode, Paul Valéry imagines metaphor as a dance that enacts the acquired meanings of a concept, "a kind of pirouette performed by an idea, enabling us to assemble its diverse names or images" (33). The link between metaphor and ideas leads Jacques Derrida in a different direction; in the discourse of philosophy, he argues, metaphor is not a figurative distraction but "seems to bring into play the use of philosophical language in its entirety" ("White Mythology" 6). For others, metaphor's influence and necessity extend well beyond philosophy. Northrop Frye, for example, sees metaphor as "the basis of poetic expression," while I. A. Richards declares more broadly that metaphor "is the omnipresent principle of language … We cannot get through three sentences of ordinary fluid discourse without it" (Frye 91; Richards 98). Kenneth Burke goes still further: "a world without metaphor would be a world without purpose" (Kenneth Burke, *Permanence and Change* 194).

DOI: 10.4324/9781003560050-1

Without purpose and perhaps without existential fullness. Denis Donoghue contends that "The supreme value of a metaphor [is] that it gives us more abundant life"—a claim echoed in a more homespun idiom by Bernard Malamud, in whose view metaphor "provides two loaves where there seems to be one" (Donoghue 71; Malamud, in Nordquist n. pag). At times, moreover, metaphor ventures beyond the strictly rational, seeming to offer an intimation of secrecy, sublimity, mysteriousness, even magic. Invoking Richards' observation that "the reader is forced to 'connect' the two ideas" of a metaphor, Max Black adds that "In this 'connexion' resides the secret and the mystery of metaphor" (Black, "Metaphor" 286). More rhapsodically, Jose Ortega y Gasset speculates that "The metaphor is perhaps one of man's most fruitful potentialities. Its efficacy verges on magic, and it seems a tool for creation which God forgot inside one of His creatures when he made him" (Ortega y Gasset 33).

Finally, an exchange from a very recent text (2024), Percival Everett's *James: A Novel*:

> "'Metaphor,' I said.
> 'That's nearly all we have,' Easter said."
>
> *(Everett 154)*

Modes of Analysis

Except to strict literalists and some others, then, metaphor is an indispensable resource of language and thought, even of being: evocative, imaginative, quasi-sensuous, world-expanding, identified at times with poetry, with literature generally, or with imagination itself. Is a compact yet thorough study of such a complex and many-sided phenomenon even possible? Previous analysts of metaphor have approached the subject by a variety of different avenues, chief among them the following: (1) A comprehensive **survey of instances or examples**, covering a variety of historical periods, cultures, and languages, analyzing representative texts, and attempting to generalize meaningfully from these examples; (2) A broad **analysis of the history of the idea**, of the many discussions—linguistic, literary, rhetorical, philosophical—of this most prominent figure of speech, from ancient times to the present. As Marcus B. Hester puts it, "one can survey the definitions of metaphor in the history of literature and philosophy and generalize from these theories to an adequate definition of metaphor" (Hester 13). The Appendix of this book (pp. 95–97) paraphrases M. H. Abrams' lucid and definitive entry on four principal "Theories of Metaphor," from Aristotle to the late twentieth century, in his valuable *Glossary of Literary Terms*. (3) An **investigation of the place or role of metaphor in different cultural contexts and systems**: in taxonomies of figurative language, in aesthetic movements and literary-historical genres, in non-literary discourses such as scientific, philosophical, or religious prose, or in legal discussions of free speech legislation—even in advertising, propaganda, everyday conversation, song lyrics, and greeting cards.

An important example of this third mode of inquiry analyzes the role of metaphor in the construction of our everyday conceptual and ideological systems. Such studies include *The Social Use of Metaphor: Essays on the Anthropology of Rhetoric*, edited by J. David Sapir and J. Christopher Crocker (1977); George Lakoff and Mark Johnson's wide-ranging survey, *Metaphors We Live By* (1980); and somewhat more popular accounts such as the many books and essays of Deborah Tannen on everyday discourse (1980s–2000s)—for instance, *You Just Don't Understand: Women and Men in Conversation* (1990)—and Susan Sontag's influential *Illness as Metaphor* (1978). Approaches like these have produced valuable results, though focused on usage and social function rather than theoretical definitions and analyses. "Cognitive" or "conceptual" accounts of metaphor, especially as exemplified by the work of Lakoff and Johnson, are less concerned with what metaphor is and how it produces meaning than with the uses to which metaphor has been put. They are therefore far less attentive to metaphor as a linguistic phenomenon than as a matter of conceptual systems.

As a reviewer of Lakoff and Mark Turner's *More Than Cool Reason: A Field Guide to Poetic Metaphor* (1989) puts it:

> The book is probably at its weakest when dealing with the tough questions of the relation of thought and language. Although generally sympathetic to the Whorfian view that language shapes thought, Lakoff and Turner fall back on the mentalist position that *concepts precede and stand outside of language, so that language only "expresses" these concepts.*
>
> *(Lemke 249, my italics)*

Much the same could be said of *Metaphor: A Practical Introduction*, in which Zoltán Kövecses focuses on the question "What has exactly happened in the past two decades in the cognitive linguistic study of metaphor?" (11). Like most scholars in the field he describes, Kövecses confines himself to "domains" that are conceptual but rarely linguistic. This is apparent from the fact that the index, and indeed the book, makes almost no mention of any theorist besides Lakoff (and Kövecses himself), or any theory other than cognitive. This inattention to language is the principal reason that the present study—which treats words and concepts, what linguists call signifiers and signifieds, as inseparable terms—devotes minimal attention to cognitive or conceptual views of metaphor. Cardinal Newman's contrasting statement of the inseparability of thought and language is as powerful now as it was in 1852:

> Thought and speech are inseparable from each other. Matter and expression are parts of one: style is a thinking out into language ... When we can separate

> light and illumination, life and motion, the convex and the concave of a curve, then will it be possible for thought to tread speech under foot, and to hope to do without it—then will it be conceivable that the vigorous and fertile intellect should renounce its own double, its instrument of expression, and the channel of its speculations and emotions.
>
> *(Newman 208)*

The question of the unavoidability of language in the analysis of metaphor was penetratingly explored by, among others, Paul de Man, in "The Epistemology of Metaphor," who on page 14 cites a crucial passage from Locke's *Essay Concerning Human Understanding* (1690):

> But when, having passed over the original and composition of our *ideas*, I began to examine the extent and certainty of our knowledge, I found it had *so near a connexion with words that, unless their force and manner of signification were first well observed, there could be very little said clearly and pertinently concerning knowledge, which, being conversant about truth, had constantly to do with propositions.* And though it terminated in things, yet it was, for the most part, *so much by the intervention of words that they seemed scarce separable from our general knowledge.* At least they interpose themselves so much between our understandings and the truth which it would contemplate and apprehend that, like the medium through which visible objects pass, their obscurity and disorder does not seldom cast a mist before our eyes and impose upon our understandings.
>
> *(Locke,* Essay, *my italics except for* "ideas"*)*

A different and somewhat more concentrated method than the three that I describe above thus entails, in addition to attending resolutely to language, (4) **Isolating an essential and constitutive feature of metaphor and following it out from a narrow and simpler focus to one that is broader and more complex**—a focus combining theory, selected examples, interpretive analysis, and consistent attention to the heart of the argument. Such an approach sacrifices breadth and range for depth and unity of focus. It analyzes "how or why the language in the metaphor means," and thus "leads to a theory of meaning of poetic metaphor" (Hester 13).

A powerful example of this argumentative strategy—intentionally far afield from metaphor in order to clarify its *methodological* pertinence—is Edmund Burke's *Reflections on the Revolution in France* (1790). Though lengthy—some 250 pages without the appendix added in 1791—the *Reflections* are nonetheless procedurally very instructive. Burke might have conducted a comprehensive survey of the French and other revolutions (see number 1 above); or an analysis of the history of the *idea* of revolution, ancient to modern (2 above); or an explanation of the place of revolution in different contexts and systems: political, intellectual, economic, religious, artistic (3 above). But for all its range of reference and allusion, Burke's withering critique of the French Revolution instead returns regularly and frequently to the conceptual, philosophical, and ideological focus of his argument: the conflict between a reliance on abstract reason alone and a respect for concrete historical and social traditions. That respect extends even to those beliefs and customs that seem and indeed may be irrational but are justified—at times almost sanctified—by the sheer fact of their historical persistence.

An early passage from the *Reflections* brings these ideas and arguments together:

> I flatter myself that I love a manly, moral, regulated liberty ... But *I cannot stand forward and give praise or blame to anything which relates to human actions, and human concerns, on a simple view of the object, as it stands stripped of every relation, in all the nakedness and solitude of metaphysical abstraction. Circumstances (which with some gentlemen pass for nothing) give in reality to every political principle its distinguishing color and discriminating effect.*
>
> *(Edmund Burke,* Reflections *7, my italics)*

In Burke's view, the Revolutionaries have torn their simplistic, abstract conception of liberty from its historical and human contexts. As the French conceive it, the principle of liberty is a ghostly, deracinated abstraction, connected to nothing around it, deprived of its concrete complexity and identity by those who ignore the circumstances and coloring that supply its true meaning, life, and actuality. "Circumstances," Burke says elsewhere, "are infinite, are infinitely combined, are variable and transient: he who does not take them into consideration is not erroneous, but stark mad; ... he is *metaphysically mad*" (Burke, *Speech on a Motion* n. pag., my italics).

To such rationalized abstraction Burke opposes the values of history, tradition, the circumstantial, concreteness—the substantiality of life as it has been lived rather than defined or reduced to abstract principle. In Burke's usage, moreover, "circumstance" means not just that which surrounds or contextualizes an event or institution but that which gives it weighty and significant being at all. Moreover, this abstract/concrete opposition informs two parallel contrasts: between the internal and the external, and the essential and the superficial. And as with "circumstances," Burke inflects these oppositions in an untraditional way, denigrating the insubstantial abstraction of the internal and championing the substantial specificity of the external, as exemplified here by the vocabulary of aesthetics and art, appearance, color, beauty, clothing, and more. Under the Revolutionaries, argues Burke, "all is to be changed":

> All the pleasing illusions which made power gentle, and obedience liberal, which harmonized the different shades of life, and which, by a bland assimilation, incorporated into politics the sentiments which beautify and soften

> private society, are to be dissolved by this new conquering empire of light and reason. All the decent drapery of life is to be rudely torn off. All the superadded ideas, furnished from the wardrobe of a moral imagination, which the heart owns, and the understanding ratifies, as necessary to cover the defects of our naked shivering nature, and to raise it to dignity in our own estimation, are to be exploded as a ridiculous, absurd, and antiquated fashion.

As in an anonymous x-ray image, human individuality is reduced to a grim and threadbare commonality:

> a king is but a man; a queen is but a woman; … Regicide, and parricide, and sacrilege, are but fictions of superstition, corrupting jurisprudence by destroying its simplicity. The murder of a king, or a queen, or a bishop, or a father, are only common homicide.
>
> *(Edmund Burke,* Reflections *77)*

In short, almost wherever Burke turns in his lengthy and fine-grained analysis, he recurs to what is for him the conceptual heart of his subject and thereby lends his argument unity, clarity, and readerly intelligibility.

The Heart of Metaphor: Truth, Falsity, Indirectness

My aim is to develop an argumentative strategy similar to Burke's in exploring the topic of metaphor by first describing its "heart" or conceptual center.

This center has two elements. The first is the distinguishing structure of metaphor as a statement of identity, an assertion—explicit or implied—that A is B, or X is Y. The traditional names for these two elements of a metaphor, first appearing in I. A. Richards' *Philosophy of Rhetoric* (1936), are the *tenor* (the familiar or conventional term) and the *vehicle* (the less familiar or less conventional term that the metaphor offers as a redefinition of the tenor):

The king is a lion.
Life is a maze (journey, fine wine, trial, bowl of worries).
Love is a Japanese Noh drama (battle, wager, dense fog, glorious dawn).
America is a melting pot.
"'Hope' is the thing with feathers" (Emily Dickinson).
"La nature est un temple" ("Nature is a temple." Charles Baudelaire).
"All the world's a stage" (William Shakespeare).
"L'homme n'est qu'un roseau" ("Man is nothing but a reed." Blaise Pascal).
"History is a nightmare from which I am trying to awake" (James Joyce).
"Ireland is the old sow that eats her farrow" (James Joyce).

In some metaphors, the identity of tenor and vehicle is implied rather than directly stated:

Down the highway of life, we live and learn. [Life is a highway.]
I woke from love, sadder but wiser. [Love is a dream, a sleep, perhaps an anesthetized or drug-induced state.]
"O wild West Wind, thou breath of Autumn's being" [Percy Shelley. The West Wind is the breath of Autumn, a wild, fierce, invisible spirit.]

This first element of the heart of metaphor entails or necessitates the second, because whatever truth a reader may find in any given metaphor, there is inevitable falsity as well. That is because every metaphor, as an assertion of identity, is a claim that one thing is another, but in the words of eighteenth-century Anglican bishop Joseph Butler, "Every thing is what it is, *and not another thing*" (my italics). Thus the reader who finds a metaphor to be true is correct, but so is Bishop Butler. Essentially, then, a metaphor is (1) a statement of identity that is (2) simultaneously true and false. Additionally, as an amalgam of truth and falsity, it is thus at odds with itself, a tensional or paradoxical structure. If such a structure invokes something new and surprising but also "something long known to us, once very familiar ... nothing else than a hidden, familiar thing," it may also prove to be an instance of what we shall discuss further along as "the uncanny" (Freud, "The 'Uncanny'" 15).

Another way of conceptualizing this dyad of truth and falsity is to see a metaphor as equating or identifying *one or more parts* of each element, tenor and vehicle, and silently dismissing the rest as irrelevant. The semiotician Charles Morris, for example, offers this formula: "A sign is *metaphorical* if in a particular instance it is used to denote an object which it does not literally denote in virtue of its signification, but which has some of the properties which its genuine denotata have" (Morris 136). More recently and particularly, in his essay "Synecdoques" Tzvetan Todorov has understood metaphor as a "double synecdoche," in which a part of the tenor and a part of the vehicle stand for the whole of each and are metaphorically identified. Thus, when Pascal claims that "Man is but a reed," he implicitly identifies the weakness or frailty of the reed with the corresponding qualities in a human being. But he does not seek a human counterpart to the reed's ability to draw water up its capillaries, or a reed's counterpart to the human ability to whistle or to wink. Todorov's is an elegant formulation, although it gains its clarity and simplicity by sacrificing the surprise, or mystery, or "scandal" of metaphoric identification. We might say that it tames in order to elucidate (Todorov 26–35).

The indirectness that characterizes metaphoric expressions—indirect because metaphors tell us what a thing is by telling us that it is another thing—is part of a larger tendency to see literature in general and poetry in particular as forms of discourse that value the oblique over the straightforward. Robert Frost remarks that "Poetry provides the one permissible way of saying one thing and meaning another." He continues: "People say, 'Why don't you say what you mean?' We never do that, do we, being all of us too much poets. We like to talk in parables and in hints and in indirections—whether from diffidence or from some other instinct" (Frost, "Education by Poetry" 719–20). Here, Frost is insisting on the indirectness or obliquity of poetry, or of literature generally, but not simply indirectness: he is tacitly honoring the particular kind of obliquity that takes us to the goal more surely and interestingly than a direct course might. Polonius, in Shakespeare's *Hamlet*, speaks of such purposive circuitousness in the business of life rather than literature: "And thus do we of wisdom and of reach,/With windlasses and with assays of bias,/By indirections find directions out" (*Hamlet*, II.i.63–5). A "windlass" here refers to "A circuit [rather than a straight line] made to intercept the game in hunting," and more generally or figuratively, "circuitous movement" (OED, s.v. "windlass," n.2). And "bias" denotes either the shape or the uneven weighting of a bowl in the game of lawn bowls that causes it to take a curving path (also called a bias), often to enable it to bypass another bowl that would obstruct it if the bowl were rolled in a straight line. A particular form of such obliquity concerns the fictiveness or falsity of literary texts—the idea being that an oblique literary strategy can at times reach a goal that a more direct strategy cannot. In Shakespeare's *As You Like It* (III. iii.16–19), for example, when asked by the literal-minded goatherd, Audrey, if poetry is "honest in deed and word … a true thing," the character Touchstone replies: "No, truly; for the truest poetry is the most feigning"—that is, the poetry that most pretends, or lies. Feigning, here, serves as the "bias" that directs language obliquely to a truth that it could not reach directly. Or, as W. H. Auden wryly generalizes in his 1939 poem, "Our Bias": "When have we not preferred some going round/To going straight to where we are?"

The poem by Emily Dickinson that gives this book its epigraph clearly belongs to this tradition of extolling an indirectness that makes it possible to communicate a truth unreachable by a more direct method. Its account of that indirectness is quite general—principally recommending a kind of text, or a way of speaking—and not limited to poetry or even literature as such. But it is clearly pertinent to poetry (including Dickinson's own poem) and to metaphoric utterance as well:

> Tell all the truth but tell it slant—
> Success in Circuit lies
> Too bright for our infirm Delight
> The Truth's superb surprise
> As Lightning to the Children eased
> With explanation kind
> The Truth must dazzle gradually
> Or every man be blind—
>
> *(Dickinson, "Tell all the truth but tell it slant," poem no. 1263)*

Truth is—like "Lightning"—"Too bright for our infirm Delight." It cannot be approached or apprehended directly but must—again, like lightning—be "eased" to us. The visual imagery—"bright," "dazzle," "blind"—points to a physical phenomenon in the case of lightning and leaves us to infer a comparable overpoweringness from a truth delivered directly, unmediated by any form of obliquity. That necessary mediation is portrayed in a variety of ways. The truth must be told not straight on but "slant"; not directly but "in circuit" (cf. "circuitousness"); its sudden force may overwhelm, as lightning may "dazzle," but that suddenness must occur (somehow, oxymoronically) "gradually." The potential exposure of all to the terrible sublimity of truth is underlined by the lightning simile in which "every man" is figuratively represented by the vulnerable "Children." And of course, "every man" may invoke another sense of "all" as in "Tell all [everyone] the truth."

More particularly, and closer to the operations of metaphor, one of the starkest ways to approach truth obliquely is to proceed along the path of falsity ("There's a 'lie' in 'believe,'" as children sometimes like to say). "Tell all the truth but tell it slant—/Success in Circuit lies." First, Dickinson suggests a semantic connection among "slant," "Success," and "Circuit" by linking them alliteratively. More profoundly, she weaves the threads of falsity right into the fabric of truth, first by activating both senses of "lies": success is to be found ("lies") in circuit, but in that same circuit success also falsifies ("lies"). Second, the necessary role of obliquity ("Circuit") is enacted in a different mode by requiring the reader to discover the conventionally correct (true) adverbial form by inferring it from the grammatically erroneous and thus "false" adjectival or noun form, "Slant." A further allusion to the falseness bound up with truth is punningly buried in the phrase "but tell it slant" for we can hear that phrase as homophonic to "but tell [i.e., measure, assess, reckon up] its slant"—that is, be aware of the necessary bias or obliquity or falsification in the truth you tell.

Dickinson's poem assumes that the apprehension of "the truth" will be overpowering, even traumatic, which suggests that this truth challenges and threatens to displace a more conventional or comforting meaning that the hearer has previously taken for truth. While the poem is about the communication and reception of truth in written or spoken discourse in general, such displacement is intrinsic to the structure of metaphoric discourse. As philosopher Nelson Goodman shrewdly remarks, "metaphorical application of a label to an object defies an explicit or tacit prior denial of that label to that object. Where there is metaphor, there is conflict … Application of a term is metaphorical only if to some extent contra-indicated" (Goodman, *Languages* 69). Which is to say that metaphoric truth (the claim that the tenor is actually the vehicle) always asserts itself against a prior and conventionally true meaning, and thus that metaphoric truth always begins under the shadow of a falsity that the conventional term initially confers on it. (For a different—linguistic—conception of the problem of truth and falsity in metaphor, see Samuel R. Levin's detailed and technical study, *The Semantics of Metaphor*, and p. 23 below.)

Our investigation of metaphor, then, begins with a founding assumption, a corollary or logical implication of that assumption, and a second implication or consequence:

1. A metaphor is an assertion of the identity of two different things: A is B, X is Y.
2. Since the two things identified are also different, a metaphor is simultaneously true and false. A is B, but A is also *not* B.
3. A metaphor's truth, consequently, is impossible to apprehend *without* its falsity.

Concreteness, Vividness, Novelty

Since this book will be exploring the relation of truth to falsity in metaphor—in particular the claim that metaphors are both true and false, and the further claim that a metaphor's truth is inseparable from its falsity—it may be useful to start with the kinds of truth or value that metaphors have traditionally been taken to make available. Most commonly and simply, metaphors are said to enrich discourse by adding concreteness and vividness, giving a sensory apprehensibility to objects or ideas, especially more abstract objects and ideas. "Civilization" and "leadership" are abstract nouns, but if, as Freud might have said, "civilization is a two-edged sword," or if leadership is defined as "jiu jitsu in disguise," both acquire a rich range of physical properties and, perhaps more important, of varied and multiple meanings that, as is often said, "bring them to life." Relatedly, metaphors are often said to confer life, vividness, or emotional power and complexity on objects and ideas dulled by familiarity, like life or death or love or misery. They *may* do so by supplying concreteness, but they need not. "Life is a lottery" or "Love is a labyrinth" owe such limited freshness as they supply to the introduction of concrete images. But the same can't quite be said of "A perfectly cooked cassoulet is a limitless joy," or "Sounds and appearances to the contrary, the entire concert was a non-existent event."

Part of the work that metaphors accomplish, then, whatever their degree of abstractness or concreteness, is a matter of freshness or unfamiliarity or novelty. In offering us what is often taken to be a similarity between one object or idea and another—the "tenor" and the "vehicle" of the metaphor—metaphors actually invite us to see one thing as another, and thus to perceive the original from a new perspective, to apprehend not just additional concreteness or vividness but also new *information* about what something is by seeing it as something it is not, or that it was not prior to the creation of the metaphor. Part of the beauty that many readers find in metaphors is just this: the beauty of a thing freshly seen—and the pleasure of that act of seeing. But there is much more at stake here: not just the qualities or attributes, new or old, of the object in question but the actual identity—or identities—of that object when seen metaphorically. Consider the famous closing sentence of F. Scott Fitzgerald's novel *The Great Gatsby*. "So we beat on, boats against the current, borne back ceaselessly into the past." This is a concrete and vivid, if sparsely detailed, image: those persistent boats endlessly driven back in the direction they endlessly strive to escape, and the medium of our lives portrayed as an undefined and indeterminate expanse of water.

But there is more than concreteness and vividness. First, the image renders us humans as ineffectual physical objects, not thoughtful agents; the sentence says nothing of captains or crew members or courses charted or sails raised or lowered. We are simply boats. And though these boats "beat on," they do so futilely "against the current." Second, the repetition and inescapability of this perpetual setback are caught in the word "ceaselessly" and reinforced by the alliterative repetition of *beat*, *boats*, *borne*, and *back*. Then there is the pun on *borne/born*, as though our being carried—borne—backward ironically keeps us from entering fully into our being and existence, from being born or reborn into our futures. Nor is there any effort to distinguish one boat—or person—from another. The plurals—*we*, *boats*—imply a common fate and a common nature, as though individual differences, identities, and strivings counted for nothing. In addition, what pushes us back is also undifferentiated: not a complex variety of weather conditions, winds, tides, metaphorically figuring a diverse array of setbacks and obstacles, but a single fateful "current."

Jaques' speech on the seven ages of "man" in Shakespeare's *As You Like It* offers a different redefining metaphor:

All the world's a stage,
And all the men and women merely players.
They have their exits and their entrances,
And one man in his time plays many parts,
His acts being seven ages.

(II.vii.145–9)

Here is another metaphor that lumps all persons into a single type: now we are actors on a stage. A concrete image but, more significantly, one that redefines our identities, implicitly replacing our customary sense of free will, voluntarily chosen courses of life, sincere ways of being and speaking, and more, with the image of us as always and inescapably actors performing in a play. A play, moreover, that we have not written, in which we speak lines that originate in an externally supplied script rather than in our own expressive choices. If we become boats in Fitzgerald, we become actors in this passage. Each redefines us, tells us that we are not what we customarily think we are but something fresh and different, if not freer or more powerful. The metaphor gives us not just vividness or concreteness or beauty but a new understanding of reality.

Metaphor vs. Simile. Redefinition. Discovery vs. Creation

It is this question of redefinition, of what we might call the ontological rather than the rhetorical dimension of figurality, that brings metaphor into sharp contrast with simile. This is a contrast that has not always been honored, or even recognized. In his *Rhetoric*, for example, Aristotle says that "A simile is also a metaphor; for there is little difference: when the poet says, 'He rushed as a lion,' it is a simile, but 'The lion rushed' [where lion = man] would be a metaphor." Accordingly, similes "should be brought in like metaphors; for they are metaphors, differing in the form of expression" (*Aristotle on Rhetoric* III.1406b, p. 205). As Paul Ricoeur generalizes historically, "In the tropology of classical rhetoric … Metaphor is the trope of resemblance *par excellence*" (Ricoeur, 174). And not only in classical thought. In traditional textbooks and classrooms of the recent and not so recent past, metaphor is frequently defined as a "trope of resemblance," in Ricoeur's words, a condensed simile, even more frequently as a "simile without the use of 'like' or 'as.'" In this view, the metaphor "Life is a lottery" is just a shorthand for the simile "Life is *like* a lottery." Both metaphor and simile are treated as forms of comparison, or resemblance, pointing to similarities between two different objects or concepts. Likewise, the metaphor "Love is a labyrinth" is understood as an abbreviated form of the simile "Love is *like* a labyrinth," and "Nature is a temple" as a compressed form of "Nature is *like* a temple." These shifting efforts to link metaphor and simile reach a kind of humorous end state in comedian Steven Wright's wry quip that "A metaphor is like a simile."

But this confusion of metaphor with simile under the rubric of "comparison" is incorrect and highly misleading. Looked at grammatically, as a certain kind of linguistic statement, metaphors are not comparisons at all, though they may encourage us to develop comparisons. Rather, they are assertions of identity, claims that one thing is another, equations rather than likenesses: Life *is* a Lottery. A *is* B. X *equals* Y. This logic of metaphor as identification implicitly informs Roman K. Jakobson's important discussion of the "poetic function of language" and in particular its "axis of selection," in which the substitution of one term for another depends on the equivalence—the identification—of the tenor with a theoretically endless sequence of vehicles (Jakobson 356, 368–9, and esp. 358). Christine Brooke-Rose, in her careful and valuable study, *A Grammar of Metaphor*, tries to clarify "the constant confusion between comparison and metaphor, found in almost every writer on the subject. As regards the thought or idea, they are indeed fairly similar … but syntactically comparison and simile present no such problems as those presented by metaphor" (Brooke-Rose 287). Some years after Brooke-Rose's analysis, the "confusion" she complains of resurfaces in studies like Andrew Ortony's "Why Metaphors Are Necessary and Not Just Nice," where the author announces:

> No attempt has been made in this paper to make a sharp distinction between simile, metaphor and analogy ... Since the traditional distinction between them is made in terms of the presence or absence of words such as "like" and "as" I fail to see any important cognitive difference between them.
>
> *(Ortony 52)*

Despite such loose claims, metaphor is both different from simile and a more radical and problematic figure of speech, introducing questions of truth and falsity, of the ontological status of objects, and finally of the stability of the world as it is conventionally known.

Our passages from Fitzgerald and Shakespeare, for example, would look very different if they relied on simile rather than metaphor. "So we beat on, *like* boats against the current, borne back ceaselessly into the past." In this simile, we are still our familiar selves; however dire our plight, we are only *like* boats, we are being *compared to* boats. In whatever direction we are borne, and however ceaselessly, that "we" designates uninterruptedly and unproblematically our familiar selves. Metaphor, however, replaces those selves with new ones, and in the process negates or erases our customary identity: we *just are* boats. And if Shakespeare had written, "All the world's *like* a stage,/And all the men and women *seem mere* players," the very assertion of what the world is like or what its men and women seem to be reinforces what they conventionally and familiarly are: the world, and its men and women. But in the original metaphoric passage, there is no world save a stage, and the men and women are always "in character": never not acting, never persons apart from or "behind" their roles. While we might concede, then, that Brooke-Rose would be correct in finding here that both metaphor and simile yoke world with stage, and men and women with players, the nature of the yoking—as she insists—is radically different depending on whether the syntax of metaphor or of simile is being deployed.

Unlike simile, then, metaphor redefines things, redefines us and our lives and the objects in our world. It offers an uncommon perspective, picturing human lives in the light of another truth than that provided by ordinary "common sense." This is to say that the metaphors we have been looking at—"boats against the current," "All the world's a stage,/And all the men and women merely players"—are not just adorning, or decorating, or making vivid and concrete the things and concepts that fill our everyday lives. They are acts of redefinition: they tell us that X is Y, that one thing is another, that seeing is always "seeing as," in Wittgenstein's phrase (Wittgenstein 196–7). In doing so, they discover or create something new in our world. In Marcus B. Hester's words, "seeing as" is "the act which leads to the discovery of the metaphor's meaning" (Hester 23; see also ch. I, "Wittgenstein's Theory of Meaning," and ch. III, "Metaphor").

We must focus, as Kenneth Burke has written, not only on the "purely figurative" use of metaphors, but also on "their role in the discovery and description of 'the truth'" (Kenneth Burke, "Four Master Tropes" 503). In a similar vein, Walker Percy argues that some metaphors derive from mistakes, but mistakes "that have resulted in an authentic poetic experience … an experience, moreover, which was notably absent before the mistake was made" (Percy 80). We should add that an experience may be "absent" because it has been repressed and now resides in an individual's unconscious. As I argue in later chapters of this book, the tension between the latent, repressed form of an experience and the form it takes when made manifest through a slip of the tongue, or a successful psychoanalysis, or a dream, or an artwork, is like the tension between the tenor and the vehicle of a metaphor. In both cases, moreover—individual psyche and metaphoric structure—those tensions may also be instances of what Ernst Jentsch, Sigmund Freud, and later theorists have denominated "the uncanny," and what Max Black terms "the secret and the mystery of metaphor" (Black, "Metaphor" 286).

As Donoghue boldly generalizes, "The supreme value of a metaphor [is] that it gives us more abundant life" (Donoghue 71). More boldly still, and widening the focus from metaphor to poetry as such, R. P. Blackmur insists on the generative and literally creative dimension of genuine poetry:

> The art of poetry is amply distinguished from the manufacture of verse by the animating presence in the poetry of a fresh idiom: language so twisted and posed in a form that it not only expresses the matter in hand but *adds to the stock of available reality.*
>
> *(Blackmur 108, my italics)*

Blackmur's final phrase, like the remarks of Burke and Percy, recalls the ongoing debate among writers on metaphor about whether the metaphor-maker discovers a heretofore-unnoticed phenomenon in the world or creates that phenomenon by articulating it. We will note here only that a newly discovered phenomenon and a newly created phenomenon add equally "to the stock of available"—that is, perceivable—"reality."

2

PROCESSING METAPHOR

Resistance and Interpretation

Schematically seen, metaphors spread themselves out between two poles according to the degree of conceptual difference or distance between tenor and vehicle. At one extreme, the pole of least difference, is a metaphor that is not really a metaphor because tenor and vehicle are separately uttered or written but linguistically identical, linked by a copula that attempts to make a distinction without a difference—a kind of bare-bones tautology. "A town is a town." "It is what it is." Such locutions do not necessarily lack meaning; one can imagine these and others, for example, being enlisted in an argument against metaphor, or against figurative expression as such, a kind of defense of literality under the banner of "We murder to metaphorize." But whatever they may accomplish in a discourse *about* metaphor, they are still limiting cases and do not really *function as* metaphors. They might be thought of as the ghosts of metaphors—perhaps the only kind of metaphor that could receive Bishop Butler's blessing. At the other pole are metaphors of maximum (at least, extreme) distance between tenor and vehicle—metaphors nearly impossible to interpret because it is too difficult to link the two terms meaningfully, or because doing so would require interpretive gestures grotesque in their laborious absurdity. These may be simple but excessively hermetic or opaque: "Lucinda is the quadratic function of lesbian Sephardic Jews." Or more elaborate: "The ocean is a rural French cooking school for Fibonacci sequences that have lost their way in the caverns beneath Hoboken."

This is to say that at one extreme, metaphoric redefinition is impeded by the excessive similarity between tenor and vehicle. Maybe not as extreme as "A town is a town," but perhaps something like "Yesterday, the waves were moving walls of water," where interpretation is certainly possible, but also constrained by the similarities (height, mass, other) between wave and wall of water. At the other

DOI: 10.4324/9781003560050-2

extreme, redefinition is rendered impossible or excessively difficult by the yawning gulf of difference between tenor and vehicle. "Squash is the C minor of racket sports." If the alliterating monosyllables "wave" and "wall" in the preceding example are too similar—both material, both inanimate, both significantly vertical, both tall in relation to the human body, both largely opaque, etc.—the game of squash and a musical key are too different. There is not enough common ground for them to be compared, whether as to similarity or to difference. The same is true of the briefly popular formula, "Color me happy" (or "sad," for that matter). There is not just a gap between color and mood but a terminological and ontological disjunction. From the point of view of metaphorical redefinition, wave to wall is an overly narrow gap. In contrast, squash to C minor attempts to leap an uncrossable chasm between heterogeneous modes of being. To be successful, redefinition must avoid becoming a form of category mistake—though see below (p. 00) for the view of metaphor as a "planned category mistake," an interesting notion that appears in one form or another in the work of Paul Ricoeur, Colin Turbayne (*The Myth of Metaphor* 1962), Nelson Goodman (*Languages of Art* 1968), and Paul Grice (*Studies in the Way of Words* 1989).

With its daring and radical performance of redefinition and generativity, then, its bold claims that one thing is another thing, metaphor does not only distinguish itself from simile. It also incurs a profound and unsettling liability by arousing readerly resistance as simile does not. For however true it may seem, and in whatever sense a reader finds it to be true, there is no denying that a metaphor—any metaphor—is simultaneously false: a non-truth. One might almost see the traditional insistence on taking metaphor to be a form of simile or comparison as an effort to evade this problem that every metaphor—but no simile—actually poses: the problem that the central claim or assertion of a metaphor is also its own refutation. We may resist a given simile as inappropriate or implausible or poorly chosen, may say that whatever this king is like, he is not like a lion, but simile does not affront us with a claim that the king—however regal or unregal—is actually *something other than a king.* As Donoghue observes, "If you take … metaphor seriously, you provoke the resistance of common sense … A simile compares one thing to another without changing either of the entities compared … A metaphor incurs resistance from our sense of absurdity": the absurd claim, say, that we are boats (Fitzgerald), or players *tout court*, actors 24/7 (Shakespeare) (Donoghue 200–1). We naturally resist this, but, having resisted it, we may be led to ponder it and, in doing so, to replace one definition with another, however experimentally or provisionally. (This topic is taken up interestingly by F. E. Sparshott (75–94) and by Jonathan Culler (1974, 219–29).

Metaphors such as the extreme examples above (Lucinda as quadratic function, ocean as French cooking school, squash game as C minor) recall a statement of the Surrealist André Breton: "To compare two objects, as remote from one another in character as possible, or by any other method put them together in a sudden and striking fashion, this remains the highest task to which poetry can aspire" ("Comparer deux objets aussi éloignés que possible l'un de l'autre, ou, par toute autre méthode, les mettre en présence d'une manière brusque et saisissante, demeure la tâche la plus haute à laquelle la poésie puisse prétendre") (Breton, *Les Vases* 148n.). That may well be the case for a poetics honoring a spontaneity that approaches the automatic ("psychic automatism"), the centrality of dreams, the subconscious, and the marvelous (over the rational), and that envisions the reader as "being limited to taking note of, and appreciating, the luminous phenomenon" (Breton, *Manifestoes* 37). For the more hermeneutically inclined reader, however, who wishes to add understanding to appreciation, and meaning to luminosity, the inescapable affront of a metaphor's claim that one thing is another thing entails a sequence of emotional and intellectual reactions. The first of these is perhaps what William Empson, citing Gustav Stern's *Meaning and Change of Meaning* (1931), terms "psychic resistance" in which "The thing [here, the metaphor] is felt as a sort of break in the flow, requiring interpretation, exciting attention and perhaps other feelings" (Empson 334). The metaphor is a "break in the flow" because it provokes "the feeling of resistance to a false identity" (the identity of the object, and/or the identity—identification—between tenor and vehicle affirmed by the metaphor). If that sense of a break is unfelt or unacknowledged—"if you merely accept the false identity"—"you may fall into nonsense" (Empson 334), which would be to accept unquestioningly and unanalytically—"Surrealistically"?—the metaphor's claim that X is Y. The following cartoon by Garry Trudeau (27 January 1985) illustrates such a fall into nonsense:

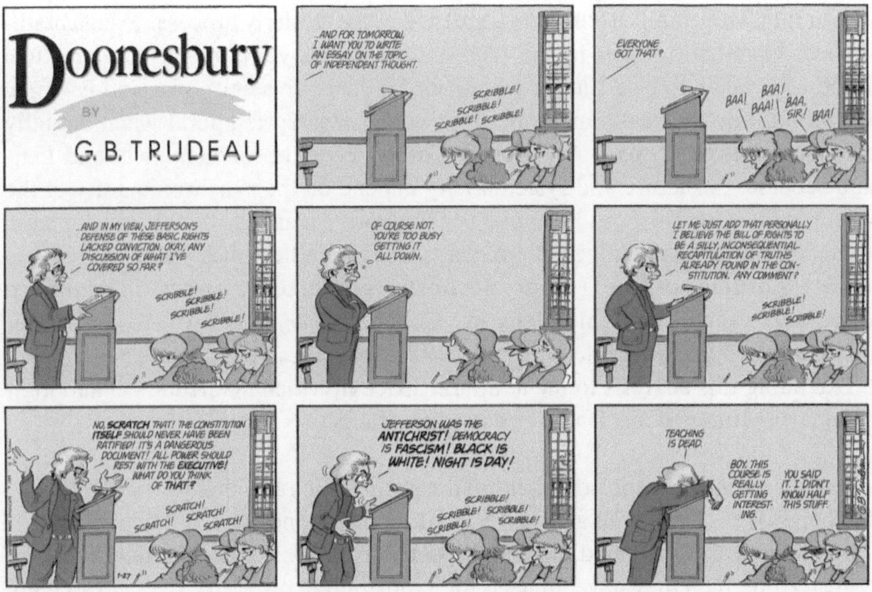

The more patient and analytic way to move from affront to understanding is to acknowledge readerly resistance to the metaphor's quasi-absurd identification of one thing with another but then to follow that acknowledgement with analytic effort. "The stimulus to interpret the false identity," says Empson, "ought to come at once from the 'psychic resistance' to it, and the combination of these two processes [resistance and interpretation] … is the only equipment we have for absorbing and starting to digest an unexpected metaphor or equation" (Empson 345). "Resistance" is the recognition of the metaphor's falsity; "interpretation" is the subsequent effort to discover the metaphor's truth in the face of that resistance. (On "incongruity" and the copula, see Brooke-Rose (113), and for further interesting remarks on the copula, see Max Black, *Models and Metaphors* (6–9—especially—and 14–15).)

Metaphor. Temporality. Education

But Empson's assertion that "The stimulus to interpret the false identity ought to come *at once* from the 'psychic resistance' to it" is a curious claim, in one sense, since it is hard to imagine how one's interpretation of a particular metaphor can occur simultaneously with the resistance that triggers the interpretation. However closely interpretation may follow on the heels of resistance, there is an almost inevitable lag or delay between them, and thus an introduction of temporality. While the copula linking A and B in a metaphor need not put A before B, it frequently does (Brooke-Rose 117–18), producing a common pattern in which the syntactic sequence moving from tenor to vehicle, from left to right (spatially, in written English), entails a temporal sequence in the readerly process. Even a mathematical equation—which in the idealization that governs much mathematical discourse is taken to be a timeless assertion of the equivalence of A and B—may be conceptually or ideally atemporal but is inescapably temporal when actually uttered or written or read. As Michael Barany notes of mathematical and logical discourse, "structure and systematicity depend on the synchronic unity of the system in question. Just as the langue is a regulative idea which makes systematic linguistics possible, the image of an ideal space of mathematics makes systematic logical exposition possible" (Barany 16; on the concept of "la langue" in Ferdinand de Saussure's linguistic terminology, see Culler, *Literary Theory* 61–2; for a fuller and richer account, see Culler's *Ferdinand de Saussure*).

Extending this analysis to the temporal space in which mathematical and logical work is actually done, Barany generalizes further:

> Indeed, a central proposition behind the purity of logic is that its truth is utterly independent of the time and place in which it is conceived and enunciated. If mathematical objects and mathematical truths pre-exist in a Platonic realm of ideal truth, then they have no need for exposition in order to exist, and so there

is a vested interest for the logical paradigm in the suppression of the actual acts of generation and transmission of mathematics.

(*Barany 16*)

Apart from the historico-temporal *generation* of mathematical assertions, any equation such as A = B, when uttered, written, or read, is a temporal phenomenon in another sense, if only because it is inevitably embedded in the temporality of speech and writing, hearing and reading.

But the temporality of metaphor is not simply reducible to the intrinsic temporality of all linguistic utterances, of the medium itself as it unfolds in time. Metaphor commandeers or repurposes that linguistic temporality and superimposes on it a narrative of redefinition. It turns an undifferentiated stretch of time into an organized duration. In consequence, every metaphor is in some sense a narrative that is a disclosure, a revelation, an "apocalypse" at some scale—not just an assertion that X = Y, but a progress from one understanding of the object to another. And unlike an equation, which—whether understood atemporally or temporally—is reversible, the identity asserted by a metaphor is in one sense irreversible, tenor and vehicle functioning not just as two equivalent quantities but also as two ends of a vector having therefore not simply a certain force or magnitude of semantic and semiotic charge but also a direction: a beginning and an ending. (But see below (p. 00) for an important qualification of this assertion.) As Frank Kermode says of the aurally equivalent sounds of a ticking clock, "Tick is a humble genesis, tock a feeble apocalypse" (Kermode 45). Sequence becomes narrative.

This is to say that the narrative dimension of metaphor is also a process of "education," itself not a simple concept. The word's etymological history displays some uncertainty about whether to invoke Latin *educare* (to shape, train, rear, nurture) or *educere* (to lead out, draw out). Further, the second term, *educere,* seems to carry suggestions of both drawing something (undeveloped abilities, say) out of a person, and leading a person out of thoughts or beliefs or assumptions that are erroneous or limiting. In short, if we educate students, we may draw forth their latent powers, or we may draw the students themselves out of one condition into another, lead them from confining error into liberating truth. In both cases, but especially the latter, the process may be difficult, even painful, since it involves not simply entering into a new realm of knowledge or understanding of reality but also learning to reject and abandon what we have—perhaps for a very long time—taken to be unquestionably the actual state of things, simply given and simply true. "In the knowable realm," remarks Plato's Socrates, to whom we shall turn in a moment, "the last thing to be seen is the form of the good, and it is seen only with toil and trouble." Or, as Milton says of the analogous moral and spiritual progress, arduous and complicated, from vice to virtue, and from error to truth, it is a course to be run "not without dust and heat" (Milton, *Areopagitica* n. pag., paragraph 9).

Plato's Cave: Blindness and Illumination, Illusion and Reality

Perhaps the archetypal version in Western literature of this journey from shadow to actuality, darkness to light, is the allegory of the cave at the beginning of Book 7 of Plato's *Republic* (Plato, *Republic* 208–11). This account of a fictional people—fettered from childhood so as to be unable to look anywhere but straight before them, and whose only reality, therefore, is a parade of shadows (cast by a fire behind them) and a barrage of echoes (bouncing off a wall in front of them)—offers a number of parallels to the illumination or education that the temporality of metaphor enacts. First, what the cave dwellers take to be reality is unreal (shadows, echoes)—a point that Plato underlines by adding that the "low wall" behind the prisoners is "like the screen in front of people that is provided by puppeteers, and above which they show their puppets." That is, the prisoners see not just mere shadows, but shadows like the stylized (and therefore "false") representations of persons in puppet shows: "the shadows of those artifacts," as Plato says, or shadows of simulacra. Second, since the cave dwellers have been fettered "since childhood," these images—or images of images—are to them what is real, what is ordinary: what is customary, normative, and therefore unquestioned.

That is why, if they were to be "released from their bonds" and freed to look "toward the light," they would not discover a realm of superior reality but would be "unable to see the things whose shadows [they] had seen before, because of the flashing lights" from the fire. Thus "pained" rather than illuminated, the freed prisoners "would be puzzled" and think that the things seen earlier "were more truly real" than the ones rendered newly visible. If forced now to look at the firelight itself, which would hurt their eyes, they would again flee to the familiar shadows that they now believe "are really clearer" than the objects newly disclosed to them. Further, if they were then dragged from the fire-lit scene and the fire "into the light of the sun" itself, they would be "pained and angry" and "unable to see a single one of the things now said to be truly real." At first confused by the appearance of real things in the light produced by the fire, they are momentarily—"eyes filled with sunlight"—rendered sightless. It is striking and significant that the path from familiar illusion to new illumination and actuality (like the path from falsity to truth in metaphor) first entails so much confusion, regression, and blindness. As will become clear, this combination also marks the operations of the unconscious and the experience of the uncanny: what Jentsch terms a "lack of orientation," and Freud "that class of the terrifying which leads back to something long known to us, once very familiar … nothing else than a hidden, familiar thing" (Freud, "The 'Uncanny'" 15).

Having come to see first shadows, images, and reflections, though, the former prisoners are at last capable of seeing the sun itself—"the form of the good"—and, recalling their former condition, they "count [themselves] happy for the change and pity the others" still confined to darkness and illusion. Thus illuminated, if a newly freed prisoner were to re-descend to the cave and resume his former restricted posture, his eyes would "be filled with darkness, coming suddenly out of the sun like that." In a thought-provoking bit of symmetry, Plato suggests that if illusion can obscure reality, authentic vision can also cloud the formerly intelligible realm of illusion. Once again below ground, his eyesight not yet readjusted to troglodytic murkiness, the former prisoner would also "provoke ridicule" among his former community. "Wouldn't it be said of him," Socrates asks, "that he had returned from his upward journey with his eyes ruined, and that it is not worthwhile even to try to travel upward?" At this point, ridicule and defensive social cohesion even begin to slide into murderous conformity: "And as for anyone who tried to free the prisoners and lead them upward, if they could somehow get their hands on him, wouldn't they kill him?" We are left with a vision of the tyrannical hold of the customary and conventional, and with the ambiguous status of the unconventional seeker after truth. After all, says Socrates, we must remember "that eyes may be confused in two ways and from two causes: when they change from the light into darkness, or from the darkness into light." There is shock at the newly revealed reality that replaces former illusion, and shock at the once familiar illusion that this reality has just replaced.

Plato's parable bears on the question of metaphor in several ways, some obvious (each is a narrative replacing one kind of understanding with another) and some less obvious. The two most prominent features of the cave dwellers, for example, are that they unknowingly live in a world of illusions, shadows, falsity, and that this world they share and know is at the same time normative, given; there is no hint of dispute about its status as reality, or of an alternative notion of how things are. Their world, that is, is at once wholly ordinary and wildly out of touch with the actual truth of things. That may not seem at first to be an apt description of the initial condition of readers or hearers of a metaphor; nonetheless, it is a dramatic and hyperbolic version of just such a condition. Hyperbolic because to encounter a metaphor is to enter a space of change and redefinition, but usually in relation to only one object or concept or class of either: "La nature est un temple" ("Nature is a temple"), or "Death is the mother of beauty," or "But, soft! what light through yonder window breaks?/It is the east, and Juliet is the sun," or "Her whole Life is an Epigram smack smooth & nobly pend/Platted quite neat to catch applause with a sliding noose at the end." Such metaphors aim to alter our notions of nature, or death, or of window-light and a young woman, or of one woman's life. They do not, like the revelations of Plato's cave, attempt to sweep away and replace the whole of reality as we know it. Thus, "hyperbolic."

But the structure of revelation or education is common to both. Recall the stages of acceptance or naturalization that Empson describes, in which a metaphor is first "felt as a sort of break in the flow, requiring interpretation, exciting attention and perhaps other feelings." Such a "break" provokes "the feeling of resistance to a false identity": that is, to the new and more or less startling rewriting of the tenor as the vehicle—of nature as a temple, for example. This moment replays the cave dwellers' puzzlement at the new reality, or seeming unreality, before them, and their instinctive recoil from it and return to the familiarity of the shadows and echoes that they had known—even though that familiar scene will itself be troubled by the revelation that has begun to occur. Having seen nature as a temple, however problematically, is it possible to run the film backward, so to speak, and see it once again as, simply, nature? At this point, if the subject does not passively and thoughtlessly accept the new definition, he or she must convert the initial "psychic resistance" into a process of interpretation that permits the metaphor to be absorbed and digested, that moves from the metaphor's falsity to the new truth it offers even in the face of that initial resistance.

And while it seems unlikely that society would seek to kill anyone who insisted on the new definition and encouraged others to share it, as Socrates suggests, it is undeniable that a common, conventional, and culturally accepted concept, "nature," has been in some small way—or to some small audience—overthrown and displaced by the upstart "temple." Recall Nelson Goodman's remark that "metaphorical application of a label to an object defies an explicit or tacit prior denial of that label to that object. Where there is metaphor, there is conflict" (Goodman, *Languages of Art* 69). Here, "prior denial" can mean simply established usage, the galaxy of actual or potential rejections that must occur in order to clear the field for the "proper" and customary term. "Reality," remarks Wallace Stevens, "is a cliché from which we escape by metaphor" (Stevens, *Opus Posthumous* 204). But if the stakes of this metaphoric displacement are higher—if it is not just a matter of seeing nature as a temple but, say, of seeing the lowly as exalted, the kingdoms and treasures of the earth as empty vanities, death as a portal to new and eternal life—then social scorn and resistance might well rise to a higher pitch, perhaps even a pitch of murderous crucifixion.

From the perspective of the new metaphor and of those readers and hearers who grow beyond its initial implausibility into acceptance and belief, what is now surprising is the *pre-metaphoric* understanding of the object. That is, the presumed falseness of the initial metaphoric assertion that X is Y retrospectively re-emerges as the falseness or inadequacy of the conventional understanding of the object; the power of that first revelation is an index of the power of the second, answering revelation. *How surprised we are reveals how (surprisingly) wrong we were.* Now it is the retrospectively viewed X (or tenor)—along with one's prior belief in it—that affronts or surprises us or grows dubious and far-fetched. From one perspective, that new reality involves more than just the vehicle of the metaphor. The sequence by which the true tenor becomes falsified as it yields to a false vehicle on the way to becoming true recalls one of Stevens' observations—that "Metaphor creates a new reality *from which the original appears to be unreal*" (Stevens, *Opus Posthumous* 195, my emphasis). As the phrase "a new reality" suggests, the invention of a metaphor is actually a two-level undertaking. The inventor imagines that X is really Y, that the tenor is transformed into the vehicle, but also that the ordinary, everyday world is changed into a world with different rules, a world in which the first transformation—of tenor into vehicle—can be possible, can reveal truth. This is, in effect, a moment of generic change, where one or another mode of realism gives way to romance, "a fictional mode in which the chief characters live in a world of marvels" in Northrop Frye's definition (Frye 367).

Samuel R. Levin makes a related argument from a linguistic point of view. For Levin, notes Richard D. Cureton, a metaphor "can be True in the world referred to by" a "higher predicate." Thus Levin claims that lyric poets intend

> *the deviant language of their poems ... to be taken to refer literally to states of affairs in the "world" of their poetic imagination.* To account for this fact, Levin suggests that all lyric poems be considered just such oblique contexts embedded under a higher sentence: "I imagine (myself in) and invite you to conceive a world in which ..." so that all deviant sentences in these contexts can be taken literally and can be stipulated True in that imagined world. In reading lyric poetry, then, Levin asserts that in order to respond appropriately to the text, readers must not construe *expressions* but construct *worlds.*
>
> *(Cureton 329, my emphasis)*

Two comments from Nelson Goodman reinforce the epistemological dimension of metaphoric figuration and its ushering in of a new reality:

> Metaphor in my view involves withdrawing a term or rather a schema of terms from an initial literal application and applying it in a new way to *effect a new sorting* either of the same or of a different realm.
>
> *(Goodman, "Metaphor as Moonlighting" 128, my emphasis)*

Far from being a mere matter of ornament, it [the "metaphorical use of language"] participates fully in the progress of knowledge: *in replacing some stale "natural" kinds with novel and illuminating categories*, in contriving facts, in revising theory, and in bringing us new worlds.

(125, my emphasis)

At this point, in a dramatic reflex or reversal, shock at the new ushers in a new shock at the old. We come to see that the falseness of a metaphor, and the startling newness it delivers to us, is really a mirror image of our own alienation from the new reality that the metaphor provides. So one truth contained in the metaphor's counterfactual assertion is that it is not false at all. And another truth is that we ourselves have previously been dwelling in and silently accepting what actually *is* counterfactual, what is false.

Origins of Truth: In the Beginning Was the Metaphor?

Remarkably, at this point metaphor opens onto a still more radical claim. When Stevens says that "Metaphor creates a new reality from which the original appears to be unreal," what does he mean by "the original?" Possibly nothing more than the immediately preceding understanding of the object: "reed" begins to cast a shadow of the unreal on "man," as does "temple" on "nature," or "stage" on "world" (Pascal, Baudelaire, Shakespeare, respectively). But "original" may mean a good deal more than that: something like "Metaphor creates a new reality from which the very *idea* of 'an original' can be seen as illusory." That is, the constructivist dimension of the new metaphor's act of renaming and redefinition may cast doubt on the allegedly originary and pre-metaphoric—the "literal"—status of the older understanding of the object. As Ricoeur asks, "Can we not hypothesize that the dynamic of thought that carves its way through already established categories"—the dynamic of metaphor itself, which Ricoeur (following Turbayne) is tempted to view as "a planned category mistake"—"is the same as that which engenders all classification?" (Ricoeur 233; see also 141, 233–4. The term and concept of the "category mistake" are usually attributed to Gilbert Ryle's *The Concept of Mind* (1949)). Or, recalling Wittgenstein's formulation, we might hypothesize that the metaphor's performance of the act of "seeing as" applies to the allegedly pre-metaphoric object as well, which now appears not as a given prior to transformation or redefinition or cognitive "framing" but as itself the *product* of a "seeing as." Its givenness or simple "seenness" recedes into the misty distance of the perpetual quest for grounding terms (Ricoeur 212; see also 235). This is to say that the initial falseness of the metaphoric assertion of identity secondarily highlights the falseness or inadequacy or incompleteness of the conventional understanding of the object, which was not just a truth—let alone "the" truth—about X but itself also an instance of "seeing as," no less than the metaphor is. The "impertinent predication" (Ricoeur 4) that is a metaphor colors linguistic and conceptual predication *as such*.

This point is made in various ways by a number of writers on metaphor. Ricoeur (in the speculative posture signaled by the interrogative mood once again) offers several formulations in addition to those quoted above:

> Could we not imagine that the process that disturbs and displaces a certain logical order, a certain conceptual hierarchy, a certain classification scheme, is the same as that from which all classification proceeds? … [C]ould we not imagine that the order itself is born in the same way that it changes?

This is to suggest "that order itself proceeds from the metaphorical constitution of semantic fields, which themselves give rise to genus and species" (Ricoeur 22, 23). Black relies on a very different (and itself deeply metaphoric) vocabulary to make a similar point: "Perhaps every science must start with metaphor and end with algebra; and perhaps without the metaphor there would never have been any algebra" (Black, *Models and Metaphors* 242). Hans Blumenberg, too, insists on the priority of the metaphoric *via* what he terms "absolute metaphors"—"absolute," explains Blumenberg's translator, in that "they prove resistant to terminological claims and cannot be resolved into conceptuality" and therefore constitute "foundational elements of philosophical language" (Blumenberg, *Paradigms* 5, 3). "Metaphorology," Blumenberg declares, "seeks to burrow down to the substructure of thought, the underground, the nutrient solution of systematic crystallizations" (5)—a "nutrient solution" that is metaphoric and that *precedes* the conceptualizations and abstractions whose growth it fosters.

In a recent illuminating exploration of this topic, Michael Ferber asks, "Do metaphors 'go all the way down'? It may be that acts of metaphorizing created the bulk of the vocabulary of every language, and if we could roll time far enough backward we could give a concrete or physical etymology for every word, however abstract" (Ferber 244). Ferber's "all the way down" alludes to a well-known and humorous anti-foundationalist anecdote told of William James:

> After a lecture on cosmology and the structure of the solar system, James was accosted by a little old lady. "Your theory that the sun is the centre of the solar system, and the earth is a ball which rotates around it has a very convincing ring to it, Mr. James, but it's wrong. I've got a better theory," said the little old lady. "And what is that, madam?" inquired James politely. "That we live on a crust of earth which is on the back of a giant turtle." Not wishing to demolish this absurd little theory by bringing to bear the masses of scientific evidence he had at his command, James decided to gently dissuade his opponent by making her see some of the inadequacies of her position. "If your theory is correct, madam," he asked, "what does this turtle stand on?" "You're a very clever man, Mr. James, and that's a very good question," replied the little old lady, "but I have an answer to it. And it's this: The first turtle stands on the back of a second, far larger, turtle, who stands directly under him." "But what does this second turtle stand on?" persisted James patiently. To this, the little old lady crowed triumphantly, "It's no use, Mr. James—**it's turtles all the way down**.
>
> *(Ross iv–v; my boldface)*

Or, as Wallace Stevens asks in "The Man on the Dump": "Where was it one first heard of the truth? The the." (See also Laplanche, *et al.*, "The Unconscious: A Psychoanalytic Study" 156: "[It] is always a metaphor, a substitution of signifiers that is found at the root of the creation of new meanings.")

Finally, if we speculatively radicalize the metaphoric re-naming in this way to cover also the "initial" naming, not only is the metaphor both true and false—so is the conventional understanding of the object. Metaphor, so to speak, metaphorizes the literal as well, and such an understanding of things, like any form of real or apparent anti-foundationalism, can produce various forms of ontological anxiety, especially to those who find metaphor and perhaps figurative language as such threateningly deceptive and labile. This situation is curiously similar to the contemporarily (and regularly) contested status of scientific truth which, for competent scientists, is both the (current) truth about A or B or C and the bearer of a future falsifiability that will at some point give way to a superior truth. That is why scientists regularly speak of hypotheses or even theories rather than simple physical truths or laws. Misreading this linguistic and epistemological convention, many contemporary religious fundamentalists err by taking the potential falsifiability of scientific truths as a sign of the inadequacy of those truths—which are inadequate only in comparison with a mythical or dogmatic Absolute Truth. But such a truth, in not being able to question itself, also *loses* its capacity to be true in any meaningful sense. Unlike scientific claims or everyday belief or the ordinary provisionality of human knowledge, dogma can be absolute and therefore comforting in a way that undogmatic knowledge cannot be. But dogma cannot be true, even if it *happens* to be true. It "cannot be true" not because of its content but because of the modality of the assertion, which by its nature skirts or forgoes any testing of claims or theories against actual situations. By its very nature, therefore, dogma forfeits its "principle of aboutness," as one scholar has humorously put it. To such fundamentalists, a metaphor is merely a secular and unstable embroidering of an available but refused ontological invariability. A remark of Robert Frost's provides a sufficient response to such quasi-absolutist thinking: "Unless you are at home in the metaphor, unless you have had your proper poetical education in the metaphor, you are not safe anywhere … You are not safe in science; you are not safe in history" (Frost 721–2). You are not safe because it's metaphors all the way down.

3

METAPHOR AND BIBLICAL INTERPRETATION

There is a chiastic reciprocity in the figure/fulfillment relationship; each, through the other, contributes to a meaning unavailable to either alone. Figural interpretation casts light on metaphor by framing tenor and vehicle as a tensional dyad of equivalent entities. This structure informs medieval Christian conceptions of the container/contained and outside/inside relationships: the swaddling (or burial) clothes of Christ and the figure they cover or contain, or the human vessel of Christ's body and the divinity it encloses. These structures, in which container and contained, outside and inside, are separate but also intimately identified, extend to metaphor and figurative language *as such*, re-describing the allegedly treacherous "externals" of figuration as not hiding or obscuring but intimately joining with the "internal" truth that they convey.

Typology. Figure and Fulfillment, Tenor and Vehicle

The dyadic and dynamic structure of the relation between tenor and vehicle aligns with several hermeneutic models, none more instructively than the system of medieval biblical interpretation that Erich Auerbach describes in his classic essay "Figura." Traditionally referred to as typological analysis or typology, figural interpretation posits a relation between Old and New Testament characters, events, and objects according to which each is a distinct, actual, historical phenomenon—say, Moses and Christ—but their relationship is not simply one of historical sequence. Rather, Moses is at once an individual character *and* a prefiguring or "type" of Christ, and Christ is at once an individual character *and* a fulfillment or "antitype" of Moses. (For the traditional and somewhat confusing vocabulary of "type" and "antitype" Auerbach substitutes "figure" and "fulfillment.") In Auerbach's words,

DOI: 10.4324/9781003560050-3

"Figural interpretation establishes a connection between two events or persons, the first of which signifies not only itself but also the second, while the second encompasses or fulfills the first" (53). In contrast to the abstraction of allegorical signification, "The historical reality is not annulled, but confirmed and fulfilled by the deeper meaning" (73). Again: "Moses is no less historical and real because he is an *umbra* or *figura* of Christ, and Christ, the fulfillment, is no abstract idea, but also a historical reality" (34). The corresponding literary form—the link with metaphor—appears in Northrop Frye's observation that "In the metaphor two things are identified while each retains its own form. Thus if we say 'the hero was a lion' we identify the hero with the lion, while at the same time both the hero and the lion are identified as themselves" (Frye 123).

This brief summary does not exhaust the implications and nuances of the figura-fulfillment relationship. Auerbach, for example (13, 15, 22), invokes an analogy with wax and seals, remarking that although Latin authors "used *figura* and *forma* interchangeably, in the general sense of form," *forma* signified "mold," and was "related to *figura* as the hollow form to the plastic shape that issues from it"—the "'imprint of the seal,'" as in this example from Ovid:

Utque novis facilis signatur cera figuris
Nec manet ut fuerat nec formas servat easdem,
Sed tamen ipsa eadem est …

(Metamorphoses, *15, 169ff.)*

(And as the soft wax is stamped with new *figurae*, and does not remain as it was nor retain the same forms, though it remains itself the same …)

The relationship between stamp and stamped seal or imprint in the wax, then, is like that between figure and fulfillment: each is itself, but the stamp is in addition a kind of prefigurer or "proleptic imitation" of the impression it will make in the wax. At the same time, the impression made by the stamp recalls but also fulfills the stamp, including its potentiality to make an impression. That is, there is a kind of symmetry or chiastic reciprocity in the figure/fulfillment relationship as each, through the other, contributes to the production of a meaning unavailable to either taken singly.

It can be tempting to regard each as one component of a single mechanism for the generation of figural meaning, though I think that is a mistake that misrepresents the character and the partial independence of each. Donoghue, for instance, who also links the structure of metaphor with Auerbach's exposition of figural interpretation, turns duality into unity in two different ways. First, he "raises the possibility that while metaphor is a double entity, the duality might be turned into a higher, richer unity" (Donoghue 84). But in the case of typological meaning, as in that of metaphor, the essentially tensional character of the structure—which depends on both the difference and the distinctness of the two components—is central to its operation. Second, after imagining the dissolution of dyadic difference into a higher unity, Donoghue envisions a competition in which the two components of Auerbach's scheme, the figure and the fulfillment, engage in a zero-sum game. In other words, if figural interpretation, in Auerbach's formulation, "establishes a connection between two events or persons—the first of which signifies not only itself but also the second, while the second encompasses or fulfills the first"—there must be a winner and a loser. "The trouble is that the 'second' by definition has the last word: to encompass is to win" (Auerbach 53; Donoghue 37). But here again, though in a different way, the essential doubleness of the typological or the metaphoric structure is needlessly and inappropriately surrendered, by agonistic incorporation here as it had been by the quasi-Pauline version of sublation in which, as Auerbach points out, the superior term "both fulfills *and annuls* the work" of the preceding term (51, my emphasis). With respect to metaphor—as to figural or typological meanings—relation, difference, and interaction must not be dissolved into simple unities of whatever sort.

That granted, it is possible to see the notion of a hierarchical relation between figure and fulfillment (and, by analogy, between tenor and vehicle) in a more complex and more philologically or hermeneutically rigorous way. Typology, in Line Cecilie Engh's formulation,

> is more than just parallelism or analogy, and goes on to establish a relation that is not only objectively real but also revelatory. Significantly, there is also a hierarchical relation, and thus not full reciprocity, between the type and the antitype: the second fulfills the first not just as the realisation of a promise, but by retrospectively establishing the true sense of the first event, without which that event cannot be properly understood.
>
> *(Engh 258–9)*

Donoghue himself, before presenting his scenario of encompassing and thus winning, offers a more moderate formulation. Because "prefiguring events in the Old [Testament] are deemed to be fulfilled, completed, in the New," he writes, it follows that "the events in the Old Testament suffer a lack that is remedied in the New"—adding that a similar structure holds true in metaphor, "where the tenor … is completed only by the vehicle" (Donoghue 32). Here, the vocabulary of "lack" and "remedied" correctly suggests dyadic structure and a hierarchical relationship, but no loser or winner.

Container and Contained

One particularly thoughtful account of the dyadic structures we are considering appears in Susan Blackburn Griffith's exploration of the wrapper/wrapped or container/contained motif in St. Augustine's conception of symbols and figuration—an exploration that bears directly on the nature of metaphor. Griffith's "Abstract" (213) is both a rich and a succinct account of her argument:

> In his discussions of figurative language, Augustine distinguishes between sign and signified. In his preaching, he hints at a deeper connection between the two categories. At various points in his sermons, he refers to symbolic language and figures as the 'wrappings' ('involucra') within which divine truth lies waiting to be 'shaken out,' like gems from a bag. Yet he has a higher regard for those wrappings than might be apparent at first glance. In Sermo 160, for example, he equates the wrappings with the crucified Christ – the humble, humiliated Saviour, too easily rejected and tossed aside. [See, e.g., KJV, Isaiah 53:3: "He is despised and rejected of men; a man of sorrows, and acquainted with grief: and we hid as it were our faces from him; he was despised, and we esteemed him not."] This type of *involucrum* thus represents the incarnational humility of God: the accessible Son of Man. The wrappings of figurative language thus connect with the means by which divine truth is mediated. The Incarnation transforms this process. This paper examines Augustine's use of imagery of wrapping and unwrapping to describe his perception of the function and status of metaphor, particularly in his preaching.
>
> *(213)*

This abstract points to the heart and the central originality of Griffith's argument. The traditional identification of the wrapper or container—as either a neutral and dispensable "envelope," a cloak or other covering article of clothing, or even a distracting and perhaps sinister phenomenon such as a diversionary concealment of precious items or a deceptive mode of obscurantist rhetoric (214)—gives way, in Christian tradition, to a very different conception of "wrapping." The Vergilian account of Cumaean prophecy, argues Griffith (*Aeneid* 6.100), of "the Sibyl 'wrapping' the truth in obscure statements ... entered into the Christian imagination as a kind of poetic justification for allegorical interpretation" (216). Tertullian, for example, connected "the wrappings of the swaddling clothes of the Christ Child with the grave clothes of the Crucified One," a connection that we find in Augustine as well. Suddenly, the neutral or deceptive "wrapper" (*involucrum*) of ancient—and modern—tradition is identified with the incarnate Christ, and the traditionally crisp subordination of outside to inside, or material to spiritual, is altered profoundly.

Except, of course, to non-incarnationist forms of Christian theology such as the docetic heresy, which holds that Christ did not have a real or natural body during his life on earth but only the appearance or semblance of one: that Christ was completely immaterial and thus the acts, events, and sufferings of his life, Crucifixion included, were only appearances or illusions. Griffith cites Tertullian's very material mockery of this sect and its beliefs when he declares, tongue in cheek—that "'there is nothing to be ashamed of in their 'Christ,' as he does not fill his diaper the way the Christian Christ does.'" This imaginary Christ, Tertullian goes on, "'neither initiated a burial shroud with swaddling clothes [*involucrum*], nor furthermore did he wallow in his own filth on his mother's lap'" (Griffith 216).

The materiality of the wrapper, then is tied to the materiality of the incarnate Christ. If Christ's assuming of mortal flesh constitutes a miraculous salvific humility, its mirror image is the material wrapping's elevation to supra-material spirituality.

The Outside Is the Inside

As the Catholic eucharist demonstrates, what had been merely symbolic materiality—lacking spiritual hereness and potency—is now a "real presence." Like a signifier whose relation to the signified ceases to be arbitrary and becomes what linguists call "motivated," the *involucrum* becomes organically and axiologically connected to and inseparable from what it contains and conveys. Griffith's account of the wrapper, and its analogy to metaphor and to figuration as such, is analogous to the idea of scaffolding. In common formulations, a scaffold, like a wrapper, and like the falsity in metaphoric identification, is pure means. Once we come upon the truth it makes available—the constructed building, or Christ's body in swaddling clothes or shroud, or Christ's divinity enwrapped by his merely human body, or indeed the truth of a metaphor—we can discard the means, take down or kick away the scaffold. But the tenor of a metaphor is not just a means to the vehicle; it is what it is in itself, even as it is also an enfolding, an anticipation, a thing without which the vehicle would no longer be a discovery but a customary and uncontested truth. The revelatory element in the figural fulfillment, the house or building, the divinity of Christ, is indeed what is most important, but the false literal truth is not mere scaffolding aiding the construction of the metaphoric house of truth. The scaffolding is both a means to *and a component of* the building. There is in it not just a usefulness but also another truth in the falseness of the metaphoric identification. That is why the scaffolding should not be kicked away. The difference between these models, and its significance, is clear in St. Ambrose:

> All this is mysterious, all this contains a hidden and deep meaning. According to your capacity the Word grows or diminishes for you; and unless you ascend to the heights of wisdom, Wisdom cannot appear to you. You will fail to grasp the knowledge of the mysteries; and the splendour, the beauty of the Word of God will be lost to you. The word of God will simply appear to you without loveliness, without glory (see Isaiah 53:2f.) … You will simply see Him as a murdered man, subject to our own suffering and weakness. He will seem to you as a word spoken by man; *as a letter covered in an envelope [in a wrapper]. There will be no glow, no splendour of the Spirit.*
>
> *(Ambrose 196, my italics)*

"In another sermon, in a striking variation on the theme," says Griffith, Augustine "describes Christ as *both the contents as well as the wrapper that is too easily rejected.* 'Summon yourself to this wrapper; pray that this might be unwrapped for you'" (Griffith 218, my italics). His dramatic valuing of the wrapper develops further when Augustine compares the *involucrum* with parables (218), and still further when he connects "the technical term *figura* with the image *involucrum*" (218). Following on this identification of *involucrum* with *figura*, we may invoke Griffith's citation of *De natura deorum*, 2.37, where Cicero observes that "Just as a shield-case [*involucrum*] is made for the sake of a shield and a sheath for the sake of a sword, so everything else except the world was created for the sake of some other thing" (Griffith 215). The same, we recall, can be said of *figura* and fulfillment, the former created in part for the sake of the latter. What is a kind of lack or incompleteness in the *figura* (figured as physical emptiness in Cicero's images of shield-case and sheath) is also the condition of the *figura*'s enabling of the fulfillment that completes the latter and thereby retroactively establishes the *figura*'s own full significance. Donoghue, we recall, says much the same of metaphor. Because "prefiguring events in the Old [Testament] are deemed to be fulfilled, completed, in the New," he writes, it follows that "the events in the Old Testament suffer a lack that is remedied in the New"—adding that a similar structure holds true in metaphor, "where the tenor … is completed only by the vehicle" (Donoghue 32). Tenor, *figura*, and wrapper each gain value from that which they foreshadow and whose efflorescence into full being they make possible.

At the same time, though, since each of the preliminary or foreshadowing terms gestures toward what it does not reveal but allows to be revealed—toward what it itself is not—each inevitably functions also as a kind of coverer or concealer, much as an article of clothing both covers and discloses the contours of the body within it. (This double office is caught in the common—and fundamentally oxymoronic—phrase, "revealing clothing," as in "To wear revealing clothing was forbidden at my school.") From this perspective, a covering or wrapper is valuable not simply because it enshrouds something of value, or because it may itself gain significance from what it enshrouds, but also precisely *because it covers*, because it does not directly reveal its "contents," because it is, quite simply, an *obstacle*—just as the traditional suspicion of rhetorical forms of wrapping and covering, of deceptive or obscuring speech, regularly asserted. In this interpretation, Bishop Butler's objection that "Every thing is what it is, and not another thing" is curiously correct. Butler, one might say, lives in a world of infinite tenors and no vehicles, of things whose ontological opacity and boundedness keep them from opening onto alternative understandings and thereby producing the unbearable absurdity, to him, of multiple and competing conceptions of what any thing is. This is not Butler's language, of course, but from the point of view of metaphoric theory, his argument can be read as an insistence on the taboo character of "another thing" and therefore on any thing's essential capacity to cover, obscure, and obstruct passage to an alternative definition or conception of that thing. The narrator of Virginia Woolf's *To the Lighthouse* asserts that "nothing was simply one thing," but for Butler every tenor is an unscalable wall keeping every vehicle obscure, opaque, invisible, unreadable (Woolf 138). How confounded might Butler have been by Swift's *Tale of a Tub*, whose narrator defines wisdom in this manically accretive and metaphoric way:

> *Wisdom* is a *Fox*, who after long hunting, will at last cost you the Pains to dig out: 'Tis a *Cheese*, which by how much the richer, has the thicker, the homelier, and the courser Coat; and whereof to a judicious Palate, the *Maggots* are the best. 'Tis a *Sack-Posset*, wherein the deeper you go, you will find it the sweeter. *Wisdom* is a *Hen*, whose *Cackling* we must value and consider, because it is attended with an *Egg*; But then, lastly, 'tis a *Nut,* which unless you chuse with Judgment, may cost you a Tooth, and pay you with nothing but a *Worm.*
>
> *(Swift 66)*

In contrast, then, to the wrapper that, according to Augustine, Ambrose, and others, must be adequately valued because of the meaning, or beauty, or glory, or splendor it holds—and which it may make available to us—this second conception of the wrapper values it precisely because it also covers and therefore protects us from an unmediated vision or truth to which our human powers are inadequate and which threatens to harm or even destroy our frail and vulnerable human being. This is one of the ways the New Testament parables of Jesus, with their persistent obliquity and indirection, have been seen—especially when they are understood as a verbal strategy to reveal truth to believers but conceal it from non-believers "so [they] can't get saved, as Saint Mark says they mustn't," in Robert Frost's mischievous phrasing ("Directive," Frost 242). The book of Exodus provides a classic instance of the danger of unmediated access to godhood (NIV, Exodus 33:18–23):

> Then Moses said, "Now show me your glory."
>
> And the LORD said, "I will cause all my goodness to pass in front of you, and I will proclaim my name, the LORD, in your presence. I will have mercy on whom I will have mercy, and I will have compassion on whom I will have compassion.
>
> *But," he said, "you cannot see my face, for no one may see me and live."*
>
> *Then the LORD said, "There is a place near me where you may stand on a rock.*
>
> *When my glory passes by, I will put you in a cleft in the rock and cover you with my hand until I have passed by. Then I will remove my hand and you will see my back; but my face must not be seen."*

This notion of a wrapper or covering that protects from the taboo lethality of direct experience of the divine presence stretches forward from the biblical era through the medieval period and well beyond. As Griffith writes, "More than a millennium later [than Augustine], a rather famous, if rebellious, Augustinian monk," Martin Luther, would elaborate on the warning God gives Moses in Exodus 33:

> Whoever desires to be saved and to be safe when he deals with such great matters, let him simply hold to the form, the signs, and the coverings of the Godhead, such as His Word and His works. *But those who want to reach God apart from these coverings exert themselves to ascend to heaven without ladders (that is, without the Word). Overwhelmed by His majesty, which they seek to comprehend without a covering, they fall to their destruction ... When God reveals Himself to us, it is necessary for Him to do so through some such veil or wrapper* and to say: "Look! Under this wrapper you will be sure to take hold of Me." When we embrace this wrapper, adoring, praying, and sacrificing to God there, we are said to be praying to God and sacrificing to Him properly.
>
> *(Luther 14–15, my italics)*

The negative connotations of the wrapper, then, and of the figurative language to which Griffith shows they are historically linked, do not constitute the full significance of either. Indeed, both figuration and wrapper should be seen as functional, significant, even essential to the larger truth they help constitute, as scaffolding is essential to the building it helps to construct. In this passage, Luther segues interestingly from form, signs, and coverings to ladders, and back to coverings, veils and wrappers. The ladder is a particularly rich symbol, recalling as it does both a figure like Icarus, who falls from his hubristic ascent, and the Tower of Babel, designed by the Babylonians not only to "make us a name," but also, like Icarus' wings, to "reach unto heaven." In Luther, however, the ladder is an emblem of the *proper* way to approach the Godhead and its majesty, while those who "fall to their destruction" disastrously "ascend to heaven without ladders" and are "overwhelmed" by God's majesty. (The story is told in Genesis 11:1–9.) Thus for mere humans, the ladder is not simply the separable, instrumental, and dispensable piece of equipment that we know from common usage but also an essential and organic part of the experience of the Godhead. All that humans may and can know safely is the compound "ladder-plus-God," a formulation that evokes the linguistic term "clitic" (proclitic or enclitic, before or after), an element of language that cannot exist except in bound form with another linguistic element: like the abbreviated form of *not—n't*—in such words as "can't," "won't," and so on. For humans, there is no God without the ladder, or the scaffold.

4

THE PERSISTENCE OF THE TENOR

Falsity in Truth

The Persistence of the Tenor

Like the key terms of figural interpretation in Auerbach, and the figural strategies of a variety of theological texts, the relationship between tenor and vehicle has been most often characterized by formulations suggesting a tensional doubleness: as a combination of the "similar and dissimilar" (Sapir, "Anatomy" 6); as terms that "are *one in that they are alike, two in that they are not alike*" (9); as a "double aboutness" (Hills, "Metaphor," *Stanford Encyclopedia*, s.v. "metaphor"); as (in Jacques Rancière's reading of Proust) "a sense of doubleness" prefatory to "a new sense of the real" (Melaney 52); and—emphasizing not just doubleness but in particular the energies of contrariety—as a "disruption," or "resistance to harmony" (Blumenberg, "Prospect" 83). "Resistance to harmony" is the phrase by which Blumenberg's translator renders Husserl's "*Widerstimmigkeit*," which is perhaps more pertinently rendered as "countervoicedness." (I offer this speculative translation against the advice of two Cornell University colleagues, both outstanding Germanists—Professor Anette Schwarz and Professor Peter Gilgen—who are in no way responsible for my obstinacy.) Indeed, in a witty if culturally outdated bit of personification, Nelson Goodman brings together not just two opposed voices but two persons in a relationship marked as much by disunity as by unity: "Briefly, a metaphor is an affair between a predicate with a past and an object that yields by protesting" (Goodman, *Languages of Art* 69). In the metaphor "Her mouth was a fountain of delight," for example (from Kate Chopin's *The Storm*), "fountain of delight" is "a predicate with a past" because it carries its own history of meanings, nuances, and instantiations, while "mouth" is an object that "yields by protesting" in that it submits itself to the redefinition proposed by "fountain of delight" even as it insists on its own pre-metaphoric identity and meaning. Goodman seems

DOI: 10.4324/9781003560050-4

drawn to romantic metaphors with a naughtily roguish tinge: "Indeed, a metaphor might be regarded as a calculated category-mistake—or rather as a happy and revitalizing, even if bigamous, second marriage" (*Languages of Art* 73). For a similar formulation in a more abstract idiom, see also Goodman's "Metaphor as Moonlighting," 29, in which he characterizes the use of metaphor as a way to "take advantage of established habits in the process of transcending them"—though "transcending" must also include maintaining the legibility of what is transcended, as I argue here. Such formulations preserve doubleness and hierarchy, a persistence without absorption of the "weaker" or subordinate or provisional term into a structure that may seem to allow it only instrumental significance. That is, the first term in each case is not conceived on the model of a booster rocket, delivering its thrust and then falling away into irrelevance; it remains an integral and persistent agent in the structure of the whole figure of speech. The "expressive labor" it performs exerts what Hills calls a palpable "semantic twist" on the vehicle. Or, to take an analogy from stage performance, an actor does not simply dissolve into his or her role or character, but persists as a person playing or assuming that role or character. If this were not the case, the performances of a single role by different actors in two different productions would hardly—if indeed at all—differ from each other.

This persistence or conservation of tenor or *figura* or first term may be described in a variety of ways. In Auerbach, we begin with a literality that potentiates a figurality that retroactively grants the literal its significative and ontological fulfillment. At one point, Blumenberg remarks that "Metaphor retains the wealth of its heritage" ("Prospect" 85). But elsewhere, as we have seen, he adopts a somewhat more sublime vocabulary of powerful hidden depths, of the archaic and primordial: "Metaphorology seeks to burrow down to the substructure of thought, the underground, the nutrient solution of systematic crystallizations" (*Paradigms* 5.) On this aspect of Blumenberg's vocabulary and philosophical stance—for example, "metaphors are fossils that indicate an archaic stratum of the trial of theoretical curiosity" ("Prospect" 82)—Robert Savage rightly remarks that "Blumenberg's contention that metaphors are historical 'in a more radical sense' than concepts, that they point the way to an occluded, subterranean realm … resonates unmistakably with … the late philosophy of Martin Heidegger" (Blumenberg, *Paradigms* 139). (Heidegger's obsession with recovering a lost—especially ancient Greek—linguistic and axiological primordiality is a major subject of George Steiner's study, *Martin Heidegger*.)

It is possible to find examples less solemn and less Heideggerian of the patterns of depth and surface at work in the structures we are examining. Consider the triad of terms "signifier," "signified," and "etymology" (roughly, history of meaning). Knowing the signifier and the signified but not the etymology of a word, we may treat the resultant opacity of the name as just a feature of conventional naming, of referring or pointing to but not otherwise interpreting. If we take "centrifuge," for example, to be just the term for a laboratory machine used to separate substances, the name will seem arbitrary and opaque, in somewhat the way that "hoover" (noun) may seem an arbitrary and opaque term for "vacuum cleaner" and "to hoover" (verb) an arbitrary or opaque label for the activity of vacuum cleaning. However, if we learn the linguistic history of each, we become aware that the separating machine operates by a spinning motion that drives the materials away from the center of the machine's chamber (*centrum, fuga/fugere*—thus, fleeing the center), and that the alternative term for a vacuum cleaner is based on a popular brand name derived from the surname of a patent holder of the invention (a patent holder though not the actual inventor, James Murray Spangler, who gave one of the machines to his cousin, Susan Troxel Hoover, whose husband bought the patent from Spangler (see *The Hoover Company*)). In both instances, the unsevered and unannihilated history of the word looks forward to its status and functioning as word (signifier plus signified, or "sign"), and that status both derives its fullness from the history and retrospectively confers on that history its identity as a proleptic generator of the word's full meaningfulness. The history (cf. "tenor") acquires a unified and encompassing name, and the name (cf. "vehicle") acquires a history, a semantic and ontological depth.

Alternatively, we may say that the vehicle is essentially and inescapably a replacement, and that its character of replacement logically requires a something for it to replace. Like the color red apart from any red thing or entity—the fiction of redness *tout court*—a metaphor's vehicle cannot exist independently. More accurately, it cannot exist independently *as a vehicle*, much as a child cannot play leapfrog alone, without the existence of a "frog" or another child or some other object—real or imaginary—to leap over. It is essential that, in some form or way, the tenor of the metaphor carry forward and either point to the vehicle or be pointed to by the vehicle, or both. Recalling the old word that Auerbach rewrites as "fulfillment," the *antitype* is etymologically the impression left by a stamp or die, and is both created by the stamp and inevitably formed by the shape of that stamp. The stamp is carried forward or is a holdover in the impression just as the tenor is carried over or is a holdover in the vehicle. Max Black describes this process of carrying forward or holdover as follows:

> I take Richards to be saying that for the metaphor to work the reader must remain aware of the extension of meaning—must attend to *both the old and the new meanings together* … [Richards] says that the reader is forced to 'connect' the two ideas (p. 125). In this 'connexion' resides the secret and the mystery of metaphor.
>
> *(Black, "Metaphor" 286. Black is quoting from Richards 93. My italics)*

And in a different idiom, Douglas Berggren argues the same point, insisting on the "conservation" of old meanings as part of the metaphoric process of generating new meanings:

> As a result of the process of metaphorical construing, both the principle [sic] and subsidiary subjects are transformed and yet preserved … [I]f the initial differences between the two referents were not simultaneously preserved, even while the referents are also being transformed into closer alignment, the metaphorical character of the construing process would be lost.
>
> *(Berggren I, 243)*

To describe this process of metaphoric construal, Berggren borrows W. B. Stanford's notion of "stereoscopic vision," the simultaneous adoption of two different perspectives. "That is to say, the perspectives prior to and subsequent to the transformation of the metaphor's principle [sic] and subsidiary subjects must both be conjointly maintained" (Berggren I 243, citing Stanford 105).

Semantic Conservation: Fielding's *A modern Glossary*

A concrete example of this process of conservation or holdover animates Henry Fielding's humorous and satiric *A modern Glossary*, which appeared in *Covent-Garden Journal* no. 4, 14 January 1752, pp. 33–8 (see also Bogel, *Difference* 160–7). Claiming that there is linguistic confusion because the meanings of several key words (and therefore concepts) have changed in recent years, Fielding's glossarist offers to translate the older, conventional meanings of these words into their contemporary signification. The main—implicit— satiric argument of the *Glossary*, of course, is that the transformation of these words is not merely linguistic but a signal of moral decline in polite English society. (Compare, in subsequent centuries, Flaubert's *Dictionnaire des idées reçues* and Ambrose Bierce's *The Devil's Dictionary.*) Here are a few examples:

GALLANTRY. Fornication and Adultery.
LEARNING. Pedantry.
MODESTY. Aukwardness, Rusticity.
PATRIOT. A Candidate for a Place at Court.
WORTH. Power. Rank. Wealth.
PROMISE. Nothing.
VIRTUE. Subjects of
VICE. Discourse.

Since a glossary is "a dictionary of obscure or antiquated words," in Samuel Johnson's definition, Fielding's most basic joke concerns the very need for such a guide, a need produced by the drift of terms from their customary meanings in a modern world that has left traditional values far behind. Not only do some words change meaning for the worse, but some concepts are reduced to words alone, indicating that the ideas and values they once represented have dwindled to merely verbal status, like "VIRTUE" and "VICE"— "Subjects of Discourse," or "RELIGION. A Word of no Meaning; but which serves as a Bugbear to frighten Children with."

If the new words had simply replaced the older ones, the *Glossary* would lose its satiric point. "HONOUR" would simply *mean* "duelling," just as "GALLANTRY" would *mean* "Fornication and Adultery." The signifieds would merely have new signifiers. For the *Glossary* to function as a satiric text, the older, conventional meanings of words must not be displaced or effaced entirely but must carry over into the discursive sphere of the newer, debased meanings. Both must be "conjointly maintained," in Berggren's formulation, and it is the tension between them that generates Fielding's satire in this work. Far from dissolving into history, the older meanings survive in Fielding's "stereoscopic vision" and make possible the newer. Drawing in his introduction on the homage that Horace and John Locke pay to linguistic usage or "Custom (the absolute Lord and Master, according to Horace, of all the Modes of Speech)," Fielding demonstrates the persistence—at least, the memory—of older meanings even into a culture and society that seem to have definitively left them behind.

In the sphere of metaphor, a similar dynamic operates. This dynamic shapes the individual metaphorist's word-making, but—as is made clear by Fielding's invoking of "Custom"—it is in no sense confined to the individual, as grammatical correctness is in no sense generated by any single speaker. A massive sociocultural traditionalism, linguistic but also conceptual, ontological, even metaphysical, shores up what we might term the "standard" notion of experience, or of the world, and this traditionalism conventionally allies with the first term of a metaphor, the tenor. The vehicle, by contrast, is conventionally the new and revisionist interloper. If the tenor in Shelley's "Ode to the West Wind" asserts or assumes that the movement of air we experience in autumnal months is the West Wind, the vehicle adds that this wind is not only "wild" but also the "breath of Autumn's being"—implicitly redefining Autumn itself as no longer simply a season of the year but a living presence that can even be addressed, not just by attracting monosyllabic vocatives like "O" and "thou"—"O wild West Wind, thou breath of Autumn's being"—but by becoming the quasi-divine spirit to whom the poem's speaker repeatedly appeals: "Wild Spirit, which art moving everywhere;/ Destroyer and preserver; hear, oh hear!" (The poem's status as invocation is also reinforced by the pun on "hear"/"here"—a calling into the speaker's immediate present, and presence.)

What the vehicle unearths is the invisible—because conventional and habitual—constructedness of what had been taken to be simply natural, exposing its conventional or "mythic" status and attempting to replace it with a newer and truer vision of the real and the natural. In Berggren's formulation, "Myth … is a believed absurdity, believed because the absurdity goes unrecognized" (Berggren I 244). Frank Kermode says much the same thing: "Fictions can degenerate into myths whenever they are not consciously held to be fictive" (Kermode 39). Or, to apply a remark of Blumenberg's to the action of the metaphoric vehicle: "The goal is to suspend the taken-for-granted character of the present, which will always seem to contemporaries to be the last word that was to be said on the subject" (Blumenberg, "Prospect" 86). "The last word" because it serves as a barrier to the innumerable *next* words—new vehicles—that might disrupt the comforting taken-for-granted character of present reality. But the boundaries between any given word and both its antecedents and its subsequent forms are far from impermeable.

St. Augustine: "Why Do We So Greatly Dread Falsity?"

As in Fielding's *A modern Glossary*, the tenor of a metaphor, like the traditional meaning of a word, is difficult to dislodge, because the givenness of the known and conventional—usage—is a major element in the comfortableness of our customary and conventional world. The new becomes familiar through repetition, and the familiar becomes "natural" when its newness is forgotten. At that point, of course, there no longer is a metaphor. The vehicle has fully supplanted the tenor and has itself become the new tenor: not yet a tenor at all, actually (until a metaphor is created), but simply the current, correct name for whatever it refers to. This often lengthy and tortuous process is what has allowed the word "oversight^1"—meaning an omission, a failure to notice—to metamorphose into "oversight^2," meaning nearly the reverse: supervision, superintendence, surveillance. Compare the first lines of a once-popular 1927 song: "I'm *looking over* [noticing, seeing] a four-leafed clover/That I've *overlooked* [failed to notice or to see] before." When the first meaning predominates, at times exclusively, the second meaning is an outlier: wayward, unconventional, and incorrect. But when, after a time, the newer meaning becomes itself conventional, the older meaning turns into an anachronism, an oddity, an error. And this transformation can tell us something about the role of falsity and truth in the constitution of metaphor.

In the case of metaphor, the vehicle is the outlier. Unconventional, incorrect, outrageous, it smacks of the fanciful, the wayward and suspiciously extravagant. To those readers who value metaphor, moreover, it is still a kind of outrage (a French theorist might call it a *scandal*); but it is an outrage such readers have come to enjoy as the source of freshness, of the imaginative, the "poetic" and daring. It may not be strictly true, but readers are able to register its poetic *frisson* by recourse to a vocabulary of the emotive, the visionary, the not strictly referential—at times, to the at once elevating and condescending vocabulary of "poetic license." From the perspective of the tenor, then, it is the vehicle that is disruptive, incorrect, whether distressingly or charmingly so. From the perspective of the vehicle, however, it is the tenor that is absurdly incorrect, whatever its usage-derived credentials, or the numerousness of its semantic adherents. Yet, as in Fielding again, metaphor retains the tenor even as it progresses to the vehicle, carries over the now-false designation that the vehicle will at once require and replace in the establishment of its novel truth. The "re-" in "redefinition" reminds us of this essential and integral iteration or conservation of what is simultaneously left behind in the drama of the metaphor.

There is not just a usefulness but also a truth in the falseness of the metaphoric identification. The metaphor's falseness is a constitutive necessity. The true requires the false; the false enables the true. Lacan makes a similar point *via* an early English slang replacement of "I understand you perfectly" by "I understumble you perfectly," which "incorporates *stumble* into *understand*." Lacan generalizes: "Understanding always amounts to struggling forward into misunderstanding" (Lacan, *Anxiety* 79). A striking passage from a dialogue of St. Augustine may help to render these essential paradoxes less counter-intuitive and more assimilable to our thinking, particularly if we keep the paradoxes and contradictions of the uncanny in mind. The figure designated "R." in the dialogue introduces to the interlocutor, "A.," "a certain marvellous thing":

> A. What, pray is it? R. What think you, unless that all these things are in certain aspects true, by this very thing that they are in certain aspects false, and that for their quality of truth this alone avails them, that they are false in another regard? Whence to that which they either will or ought to be, *they in no wise attain, if they avoid being false.* For … how would a picture, for instance, be a true picture, unless it were a false horse? Or how could there be in a mirror a true image of a man if it were not a false man? *Wherefore, if it avails some things that they be somewhat false in order that they may be somewhat true; why do we so greatly dread falsity, and seek truth as the greatest good?*
>
> (Augustine n. pag.)

5

THE DECLINE OF LITERAL TRUTH AND REFERENCE

Renaissance Answers to Plato

The central issue of falsity and truth applies to whole works and not just to figures of speech such as metaphor. Works we call literary, whether poetry, fiction, drama, or other forms, raise persistent questions of fictionality and truth, and of the relations between them. Indeed, there is a lengthy tradition of writers attempting to explain how a text we regard as fictional can nonetheless make available to us one or another kind of truth. In the English Renaissance, such writers were frequently attempting to answer the charge that poetry is, in one way or another, immoral: a charge energetically developed in the writings of Stephen Gosson (*The Schoole of Abuse*, 1579) and others. That charge, in turn, traces back to Plato and the tradition of distrusting poetry as a mode of discourse dangerously untrue though perhaps very beautiful. Plato feared that poetry "nurtures and waters" the passions, thereby fostering irrationality and even the destruction of civic order. In consequence, he says that if a poet appears in a community and offers to recite his verses, "We would bow down before him as someone holy, amazing, and pleasing." And so, "We would anoint his head with perfumes, crown him with a woolen wreath, and send him away to another city." Why? Because all poetry "is likely to corrupt the mind of those of its hearers who do not have the knowledge of what it is really like as a drug to counteract it" (Plato, *Republic* 398a, 606d, 595b; pp. 311, 79, 279; see also Mitsi; Matz; and Wimsatt & Brooks, ch. 9).

As we have seen (Chapter 1), nearly two thousand years after Plato's *Republic*, the character Touchstone in Shakespeare's *As You Like It* offers a more complex and sophisticated formulation. When asked if poetry is "honest in deed and word … a true thing," he replies: "No, truly; for the truest poetry is the most feigning"—that is, the poetry that most pretends. In addition to the Platonic tradition of

DOI: 10.4324/9781003560050-5

poetic distrust, then, there is a counter-tradition that rejects the notion that poems are simply false and at times also rejects the further assumption that the true and the false are necessarily at odds. Some writers in this counter-tradition even argue that poetry is a mode of discourse whose value not only coexists with but *is dependent on* its falsity or fictionality, that it belongs to a separate imaginative and frequently idealizing sphere. Sir Francis Bacon contrasts reason and poetry in this way: "reason doth buckle and bowe the mind unto the Nature of things," while poetry "doth raise and erect the Minde, by submitting the shewes of things to the desires of the mind … Therefore it was ever thought to have some participation of divinesse." And Sir Philip Sidney argues that

> the poet, disdaining to be tied to any such subjection, lifted up with the vigor of his own invention, doth grow, in effect, into another nature … [H]e goeth hand in hand with nature, not enclosed within the narrow warrant of her gifts, but freely ranging within the zodiac of his own wit. Nature never set forth the earth in so rich tapestry as divers poets have done … her world is brazen, the poets only deliver a golden.

Note that these last six words may be taken in two different though compatible senses: *the poets deliver only a golden world*, or *only the poets deliver a golden world*. (See the discussion and representative texts in Wimsatt and Brooks 171–2.)

Fictional Truth: Creation, Consciousness, Being

Modern versions of this Renaissance insistence on the special character of fictionality in poetry or other literary modes take a variety of forms. A very late development of this tendency to liberate poetry from everyday notions of truth and plausibility appears in an essay by Paul de Man that works to free literary texts from the burden of referentiality altogether, though the essay—at the risk of some question-begging—does not indicate how we are to distinguish literary from nonliterary texts (de Man, "Crisis" 53–4). There is, as we have noted, the regular and functional uncertainty whether producers of metaphor discover fresh dimensions of experience or create them. As Max Black puts it, "It would be more illuminating in some of these cases to say that the metaphor *creates* the similarity than to say that it formulates some similarity *antecedently* existing" (Black, "Metaphor" 284–5). Like some other writers on metaphor, Black treats the discovery/creation dyad as what W. B. Gallie terms an insoluble or irreducible or "essentially contested" concept—like nature/nurture, or psychic state/brain chemistry. In a much expanded philosophical context of epistemological modes of representation, Ernst Cassirer offers a related formulation of discovery as creative construction. Here, the mind does not mirror reality but produces it:

> From this point of view, myth, art, language and science appear as symbols; not in the sense of mere figures which refer to some given reality by means of suggestion and allegorical renderings, but in the sense of *forces each of which produces and posits its own reality* … Thus the special symbolic forms are not imitations, but *organs* [Cassirer's italics] of reality, since it is solely by their agency that anything real becomes an object for intellectual apprehension, and as such is made visible to us.
>
> *(Cassirer 8, first italics mine)*

Cassirer's shift from representation to constitution, "imitations" to "organs," is obliquely echoed by Winifred Nowottny in a discussion of metaphor and poetic structure in which Cassirer's "forces each of which produces and posits its own reality" become metaphors that are "deliberate fabrications":

> Current criticism often takes metaphor *au grand sérieux*, as a peephole on the nature of transcendental reality, a prime means by which the imagination can see into the life of things; this attitude makes it difficult to see the workings of those metaphors which deliberately emphasize the frame, offering themselves as deliberate fabrications, as a prime means of seeing into the life not of things but of the creative human consciousness, framer of its own world.
>
> *(Nowottny 87)*

Another strand of modern theorizing brackets questions of truth and falsehood, reality and fiction, by viewing metaphor not as a clarification or redefinition of an entity's meaning and significance but principally as a realization of the entity's essential nature. As Walker Percy asks, "Is it the function of metaphor merely to diminish tension, or is it a discoverer of being?" Contrasting the theoretical (that is, philosophical) approach to metaphor with the critical (that is, literary) approach, Percy generalizes: "If the theorist is insensitive to the beauty of metaphor, the critic is insensitive to its ontology" (Percy 86, 82). What is at stake here is concern for the essential nature or "whatness"—not the truth or meaning—of an object: its "inscape," to use the language of Gerard Manley Hopkins that Percy occasionally borrows. "Inscape" refers to an object's internal, individual, and singular nature, and Percy takes his title, "Metaphor as Mistake," from Southern regional linguistic errors such as calling the Blue Darter Hawk a Blue Dollar Hawk, or a Seeburg automatic coin record player a seabird—errors that, in their deviation from the conventional terms, don't just substitute an incorrect term for the correct one but also shift the focus from naming, classification, truth, and description to the ontological dimension of literary representation. For Percy, the wrongness or falsity of the particular term discloses this dimension in something of the same way that the wrongness of a metaphoric vehicle discloses the heretofore unapprehended being of the metaphor's tenor. And, since this study will soon turn to psychoanalysis and the concept of the uncanny, we should note that the revelatory "mistake" in Percy's argument functions somewhat as the symptomatic "slip of the tongue" does in Freudian psychoanalysis—as an "error," but a revelatory error. Further, the coexistence of error and truth in such slips (and in parapraxes generally) also brings into view the oxymoronic structure of the Freudian uncanny, which—in Katherine Withy's concise formulation—"destabilizes the realm of the familiar," as does the structure of metaphor (Withy 216).

Percy's focus on physical objects such as the bird and the jukebox rather than on concepts is also part of the rhetoric of his concern with metaphor and ontology: a way of implying that what metaphor offers us is not just an improved linguistic or conceptual grasp of the object but a new apprehension of its being and nature. And as we have seen, Blackmur also insists on the presence, thingness, and being of what genuine poets deliver: "language so twisted and posed in a form that it not only expresses the matter in hand but adds to the stock of available reality" (Blackmur 108). "Twisted," "posed," "form," "matter in hand," "adds to the stock," "available": most of these words and phrases carry a distinctly material sense, and sometimes an overtone of fabrication or manufacture, suggesting that genuinely artful poetry provides us not just with meanings and language but with ontologically dense and numerable ("adds to the stock") objects, quasi-things. This vocabulary suggests as well that, as in Percy's essay, the singular gift of certain kinds of language is not an enhanced set of descriptions and definitions but an enlargement of modes of being—and thereby of entityhood itself. This rhetoric of materiality also appears in the Renaissance texts we have looked at—as the vocabulary of "rich tapestry" and of worlds "brazen" and "golden" suggests—and in much earlier texts, such as Horace's "Exegi monumentum aere perennius": "I have built a monument [i.e., *Horace's own poetical works*] more lasting than bronze" (Horace, Odes III. 30).

The Construction of the Real: Literary Form and Back-Formation

The development that I am tracing involves the gradual weakening of the criterion of referential accuracy in the reception of poetry and of other literary forms as well—extending (perhaps surprisingly) even to the realistic novel. Ian Watt, deploying the term "formal realism," declares in 1957 that "The novel's realism does not reside in the kind of life it presents, but in the way it presents it" (Watt 11). As we have seen, other standards such as ideality and idealization—Frye's Romance mode "in which the chief characters live in a world of marvels" (Frye 367)—fullness of being, the invention of new forms of experience or reality, the valuing of fictionality as such, have gradually transformed the question "Is it true?" into something like "Is the text's presentation or invention or production of truthfulness significant and satisfying?" This transformation is what allows David Lodge to isolate what he terms the "profound paradox at the heart of literary language … that the imaginative writer creates what he describes. It follows from this that every imaginative utterance is an 'appropriate' symbolization of the experience it conveys, since there is no possible alternative symbolization of 'the same' experience" (Lodge 62).

Reference in literature can also be understood on the model of what linguists term "back-formation," the creation of a supposedly more primitive form of a word *after* the word itself has entered the lexicon (as I have argued in *New Formalist Criticism* 91–3). Thus, on the erroneous but common assumption that verb-forms precede noun-forms, whether as historically prior or as somehow linguistically more basic or primitive, the historically later verb-form is presented as anterior to the actually earlier noun-form. Given the noun "liaison," *presumed* to be a secondary or derivative form, we produce the verb "liaise"; ditto with "burglar" and "burgle," or "enthusiasm" and "enthuse." The mechanism is analogous to the "prequel," in which narrative B is produced later than narrative A but tells a story of events preceding narrative A. The same is true of literary texts and the allegedly antecedent experiences on which they "report." Experiences or events that a poem treats as true or real and as preceding its writing ("I wandered lonely as a cloud," "I placed a jar in Tennessee,/And round it was, upon a hill") are in fact generated by the poem itself. The actual and factual are made available by the fictional and false. Which is to say that the literary road to truth seems to lead toward something other than reference, referentiality, and verifiability, and that it does so in the frank recognition that this road is paved with fictionality, with untruth, with falsity.

6

POEMS AS METAPHORS

To Truth through Fiction

Impossible Speakers, Poetic Truths

The model of metaphor in which falsity or fictionality is essential to the production of truth can be extrapolated to entire texts whose truth and power emerge from a founding counterfactual premise. Monroe Beardsley writes that "A metaphor is a miniature poem" (Beardsley 144). Perhaps we can reverse this remark and operate under the speculative assumption that a poem is a full-size or unreduced or expanded metaphor—a "speculative assumption" in Hans Vaihinger's sense of heuristic procedures that "appear to be consciously false assumptions … which are intentionally thus formed in order to … reach the goal of thought by roundabout ways and bypaths" (Vaihinger xlvi–xlvii). It is instructive, for example, to focus on a sub-class of works that are not simply fictional but that also foreground their unmistakable fictionality by creating speakers and dramatic situations that are, in terms of ordinary reality, impossible. The grounding assumption of each text is thus inescapably "false." An example of this sort of poem is Craig Raine's "A Martian Writes a Postcard Home," in which a Martian attempts to explain what he has discovered after spending some time on earth among humans. The false premise of the poem, of course, is that Martians exist, speak English, have traveled to earth, write postcards, and so on. The truth is the postcard's fresh look into the oddity not of Martian but of human behavior, seen from an alien perspective—a perspective that is naïve, unmystified, and decidedly "unembedded," to borrow a recent journalistic term.

Another version of this strategy appears in the prose "it-narratives" that flourished (modestly) in the later eighteenth century and after. In these, an inanimate object, occasionally a pet, is the impossible principal narrator, and one effect is the defamiliarized and sometimes satiric view of human life that is provided by such

DOI: 10.4324/9781003560050-6

a non-human narrator. Prominent examples include Charles Johnstone's *Chrysal; or, the Adventures of a Guinea* (1760–65), and *The History of a Pin, as Related by Itself* (1749, by "Miss Smythies")—the latter of which shrewdly explores instances of mechanization in human behavior such as manufactured or feigned emotions, thereby thematizing the doubleness of narrator and dramatic situation (see the illuminating and pioneering discussion in Mark Blackwell's *The Secret Life of Things: Animals, Objects, and It-Narratives in Eighteenth-Century England*). An interesting and racy variation is provided by Diderot's 1748 novel *Les Bijoux indiscrets* (*The Indiscreet Jewels*), in which a genie presents a sultan with a magic ring which, when rubbed and pointed at a woman's "jewel" (genitalia), compels the woman's sex to speak of its—and thus its possessor's—erotic adventures.

There are also poems spoken by animals. In Ted Hughes's "Hawk Roosting," the hawk displays a kind of narcissism that the poem allies with the bird but that also hints at the raw primitiveness of human self-centeredness. Here are just a few lines:

> My feet are locked upon the rough bark.
>
> It took the whole of Creation
> To produce my foot, my each feather:
> Now I hold Creation in my foot
>
> Or fly up. And revolve it all slowly—
> I kill where I please because it is all mine.
>
> *(Hughes 68)*

On the one hand, we recognize that the speaker can't be an introspective talking hawk so is most likely a human pretending to be a hawk. On the other hand, we may explore the hawk's utterance and attitude in itself, as what a hawk *might* think or say if somehow granted the powers of human consciousness and human speech. This is of course a grossly anthropomorphic simplification of the problem; as Wittgenstein famously remarked, "Wenn ein Löwe sprechen könnte, wir könnten ihn nicht verstehen" ["If a lion could talk, we wouldn't be able to understand it"] (Wittgenstein 225). And there is the further implication that a human might be able to speak for a hawk because a kind of feral sharing can render humans no less simple, rapacious, and self-absorbed than birds of prey. Whatever meanings and truths we derive from this text, though, are all based on the impossibly false narrative situation in which the hawk speaks.

First Person Deceased: Jarrell's Ball Turret Gunner

A different "impossible" speaker narrates Randall Jarrell's startling—even distressing—five-line poem of 1945, "The Death of the Ball Turret Gunner," the premise of which is inescapably fictive:

> From my mother's sleep I fell into the State.
> And I hunched in its belly till my wet fur froze.
> Six miles from earth, loosed from its dream of life,
> I woke to black flak and the nightmare fighters.
> When I died they washed me out of the turret with a hose.

Jarrell supplies an explanatory note:

> A ball turret was a plexiglass sphere set into the belly of a B-17 or B-24, and inhabited by two .50 caliber machine-guns and one man, a short small man. When this gunner tracked with his machine-guns a fighter attacking his bomber from below, he revolved with the turret; hunched upside-down in his little sphere, he looked like the foetus in the womb. The fighters which attacked him were armed with cannon firing explosive shells. The hose was a steam hose.
>
> *(Jarrell 144; the prose note is on 8)*

The poem depicts the gunner as continually entrapped in one or another sort of bubble. He is in the womb, he falls into a second "womb" (the belly of the State), he is in a ball turret, he is captive to and then freed from earth's "dream of life." The only "birth" he experiences is waking to "black flak" and "nightmare fighters." From one womb to another womb, and from a sleep to a dream to a nightmare: he wakes at or shortly before the moment of his death and seems to experience no authentic life. Finally, reduced from personhood to mere matter, he is "washed out of the turret with a hose." (The words grimly echo a military phrase for failing to complete flight school or other training programs successfully: to "wash out.")

What is impossible—false—of course is that this entire experience is narrated by the deceased gunner himself. Why make that poetic choice? Much of the horror, after all, would have been conveyed if the poem had been written and spoken in the third person, by an omniscient and unidentified speaker, as the title is: "From his mother's womb, he fell into the State," "When he died they washed him out," and so on. Why risk diminishing the painful seriousness of the gunner's plight with a fanciful act of ventriloquism that pretends he is posthumously describing his experience? Or, in the language of this study's inquiries, what otherwise inaccessible truth is made available by means of the fiction or untruth of the dead man's speech? There is, first, the undeniable vividness and immediacy of the speaker-protagonist's direct address to readers. Additionally, to speak *for* and therefore *as* the gunner is for the poet to engage in an act of identification with him, to articulate what he might have been feeling and to pay tribute to that otherwise inaccessible inner life. Lastly, the fusion of speaker and gunner into a figure at once alive and dead reminds us that the principle of death always inhabits the living as well as the dead, that death and life are not as distinct as we might imagine, or wish (see Dylan Thomas' *The Force That Through the Green Fuse Drives the Flower*). Only by imagining himself as the dead gunner can the poet articulate the knowledge that death alone makes available.

Such a reminder of mortality recalls a particular kind of epitaph, the conventional monitory text that Debra Fried terms an "iterative gravestone inscription of the 'Halt, traveler' variety," which frequently begins with the Latin phrase, "Siste, viator"—"Stay, traveler"— and then delivers the message the traveler is supposed to read and ponder (Fried 615). Here is a typical example:

> Remember me as you pass by,
> As you are now, so once was I,
> As I am now, so you must be,
> Prepare for death and follow me.
>
> *(Pierson 66)*

Fried (617) cites a similar verse from a Quaker gravestone:

> What thou art reading o'er my bones
> I've often read on other stones
> And others soon shall read of thee
> What thou art reading now of me.

The pause urged on the traveler can be taken symbolically as well as literally. It is a momentary suspension of the traveler's present journey, after which that journey will be resumed, but it also prefigures that final stop on life's journey when death will bring all movement to a halt. Thus the traveler's pause is a contemplation—but also a rehearsal—of that future and final pause. As Fried summarizes early in her subtle discussion:

> Epitaphs make us see ourselves as doubles—perhaps incomplete or imperfect doubles—of the dead, as living dead, as readers awaiting our epitaphs … Instructing us through mirroring lines to use the gravesite as our own mirror, epitaphs ask us to recognize ourselves in them.
>
> *(617)*

Moreover, the poet's identification with the dead ball turret gunner, who is able to speak only by means of a convention like that of these epitaphs, is made more poignant by the fact that, prior to his death, the gunner has been allowed no voice. In a sense, the poet's fictive impersonation grants the gunner not just a voice but a life—however brief—that stands in for the one he was denied. None of this (imagined) insight into the consciousness and plight of the gunner would have been possible without the initial decision to speak for and as another person.

But there is a still more troubling dimension to the poem. Consider these two lines:

> Six miles from earth, loosed from its dream of life,
> I woke to black flak and the nightmare fighters.

"Loosed" is a curious word in this context. At first, it may seem to describe a snatching away from the earth that leads to the death of a young soldier. But since the word actually means "released," "set free," "liberated," it suggests that the gunner's exile into sky and death may be a kind of gift, a liberation from the false dream of life. Similarly, the phrase "nightmare fighters" may mean "fighters as terrible as those a nightmare produces," but syntactically it can also mean "fighters of—that is, *against*—nightmares." The two lines together suggest that the poem is performing a radical, demystifying transformation of everyday values. In this new view, the real nightmare is the deceptive dream of life that surrounds and comforts earthly women and men. ("My mother's sleep" may refer not simply to a sleep that is the mother's and perhaps the foetus' but also to the mother's normatively somnolent and mystified "dream of life.") Karl Marx called religion the "opium of the people"; here, faith in life may be understood as the opium of the quotidian earthbound, the living, much as, in Kirkegaard's oft-quoted phrase, "unconscious despair" is "the worst form of despair."

Correspondingly, if what the fighters actually destroy or displace is the dream-nightmare of a deceptive earthly fantasy, the implication is that "black flak and the nightmare fighters" are the underlying truth of our experience not a horrid hallucination but a grim reality that we "wake" to, not from. By implication, if earth's "dream of life" is actually a fiction concealing a nightmare and that nightmare is as close as the living get to the actual truth of things, we approach an inversion of the categories of life and death. The poem's posthumous narration implies that only those who face and finally enter the realm of death can see and say the truth of human experience. But since an actual victim cannot speak—dead men tell no tales—the fiction or untruth of the poem's narration is the only conceivable way of articulating what the poet believes but could not confirm without dying (at which point he would not be able to confirm or say anything at all). In short, the fiction of a posthumous speaker makes possible a fresh truth that could not have been discovered without it. The poem is thus a kind of anti-revelation: a wresting from horror the insight that what is there is horror.

Such distressing revelations appear elsewhere in Jarrell. In "90 North," for example, a poem that does not depend on an impossible narrator, he writes (again in the first person) of reaching the North Pole and discovering that this goal and zenith is indistinguishable from the inescapability of descent and loss: "I stood at the northern pole/... Turn as I please, my step is to the south." Here, there is no life-affirming wisdom, no redemption of pain by knowledge as in classical tragedy's Aristotelian *anagnorisis*. There is nowhere to go but down:

I see at last that all the knowledge
I wrung from the darkness—that the darkness flung me—
Is worthless as ignorance: nothing comes from nothing.
The darkness from the darkness. Pain comes from the darkness
And we call it wisdom. It is pain.

(Jarrell 113–14)

Just as the ball turret gunner is loosed from earth's "dream of life," the speaker of "90 North" is crowded "out of the ignorant darkness" (27), a state identified with "childish night" and sleep (1–8), and with "that warm world" (18) which is also "that Cloud-Cuckoo-Land" (20)—the repeated deictic "that" signaling both the temporal distance of the past and the otherness of its false and fantasmatic consolations. The two poems share a fascination with the discoveries thrust on solitary individuals in extreme situations and juxtapose ordinary conceptions of meaningfulness with the emptiness that lies beneath them. "90 North" reinforces the thematic importance to Jarrell of what might be called insight at the end of the line: moments in which awareness or revelation comes up against the dead end of nothingness, or of insight's own vacuity and uselessness:

I woke to black flak and the nightmare fighters.
When I died they washed me out of the turret with a hose.
* * * *
... nothing comes from nothing.
The darkness from the darkness. Pain comes from the darkness
And we call it wisdom. It is pain.

(My phrase, "insight at the end of the line," derives somewhat obliquely from Neil Hertz's rich collection, *The End of the Line: Essays on Psychoanalysis and the Sublime*, especially 217–19, 258 n.2.)

"The Death of the Ball Turret Gunner" thus aligns itself with the structure of metaphor, and with the metaphoric enabling of truth by falsehood or fiction on the models of Raine's Martian, or Hughes's hawk, or the coins and pins that recount their stories in it-narratives, or the tattle-tail "bijoux" of Diderot's novel. To generalize somewhat schematically and reductively: false stands to true as earth's "dream of life" stands to "black flak and the nightmare fighters"; as the fiction of the speaking gunner stands to the otherwise unavailable truth of human experience as horror at the moment of death; *and as the fiction of metaphor's tenor stands to the truth of its vehicle*—that is, the new truth of the vehicle that emerges as it displaces the conventional and seeming truth of the tenor, managing at last, in Blumenberg's formulation once again, "to suspend the taken-for-granted character of the present" (Blumenberg, "Prospect" 86).

7

THE DOUBLE TRANSIT OF METAPHOR

Metaphor and the Uncanny

The Double Transit of Metaphor

To the series of paired terms above we can add another that foregrounds the experience of the reader or observer: self and other. A hypothetical reader's movement from tenor to vehicle in processing a metaphor is also, in a sense, a progression from self to other. As I have suggested earlier, every metaphor is in some sense and at some scale a narrative that is a disclosure, a revelation, an unfolding scene of instruction—not just an assertion that X = Y but a progress from one understanding of the object to another. The tenor is a part of the reader's and the culture's normative and internalized understanding of experience: for example, "Life." The vehicle, by contrast, is comparatively foreign to this context, as yet unassimilated, in some sense "other": for example, "a bowl of cherries." Even in a hackneyed example like this one, it is important not to minimize the transformative power of the arc from tenor to vehicle—as Donoghue somewhat surprisingly does. He speaks of metaphor's "impulse to escape from the world, and especially from the importunity of objects, things, and faces," and further claims that this impulse "is best fulfilled by putting another form of discourse in place of reference. The strongest such form is prophecy" (Donoghue 204). Donoghue's view derives in part from Wallace Stevens' conception of metaphor as a way of mitigating the existential weight and ontological brashness of the world, as in his poem "The Motive for Metaphor." But Donoghue gives away too much of metaphor's linguistic power by reassigning it to the language of the prophetic, and he goes still further when he proclaims that rhetoric in general "is a glorious failure, and the cry of metaphor is doomed: we can't, after all, change the world by finding names

DOI: 10.4324/9781003560050-7

for things" (Donoghue 184). This rash rejection first of metaphor's engagement with the actual world and then of rhetoric altogether entails the disempowering of metaphor and thus of its ability to deliver either an enlarged vision of "available reality" or a deepened sense of an object's ontological weight. Claims like these run directly counter to the views of (among many others) Kenneth Burke, who sees metaphors and other tropes as instruments of perspective, cognitive and ontological, and consequently maintains that "characters possess degrees of being in proportion to the variety of perspectives from which they can with justice be perceived" (Kenneth Burke, Appendix D, "Four Master Tropes," 503). That "variety of perspectives" cannot be achieved if we exchange the metaphorics of the text for an extra-worldly mode of discourse such as prophecy.

Moreover, the ostensibly demystified claim that rhetoric is a failure because "we can't, after all, change the world by finding names for things" seems to be true only in the context of a naïve empiricism or a faith in fixed essences or both. Seeing is, as Wittgenstein asserted, "seeing as"; what we see is altered by what we see it *as* which in turn alters what we call it, and vice versa. Wittgenstein explores this issue, in part by examining unresolvably ambiguous visual images like the well-known duck-rabbit drawing in his *Philosophical Investigations*, an image—titled "Kaninchen und Ente" ("Rabbit and Duck")—that first appeared in the 23 October 1892 issue of *Fliegende Blätter* (http://diglit.ub.uni-heidelberg.de/diglit/fb97/0147?sid=8af6d821538a1926abf44c9a95c40951&zoomlevel=2; https://commons.wikimedia.org/wiki/File:Canard-lapin_retouché.jpg):

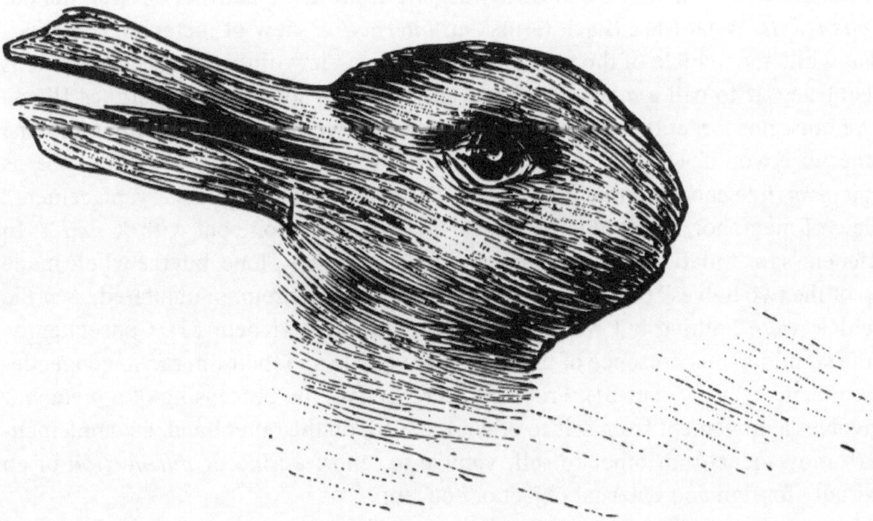

And there is no way around seeing it as *something.* "If a thing is a thing at all," as W. K. Wimsatt once remarked, "it's a certain *kind* of thing" (graduate seminar discussion, "Theories of Poetry," Yale University, 1967).

To change the names of things is therefore, whether trivially or substantially, to change those things and therefore the world that is their context. This fact is evident even in prosaic non-literary discourse. Pluto was a planet, then more recently a non-planet, then still more recently a dwarf planet. Certain American citizens are in some contexts nationalist patriots but in others White supremacists. Alcoholism is to some a disease, to others a moral failure, to still others a fictional term for a non-existent condition. And the nation's principal internal conflict has at different times and places been denominated the Civil War, or the War for Abolition (or against Slavery), or the War for Southern Independence, or the War of Northern Aggression. Even—more startlingly still—a war in "defense of constitutional rights, … as much a struggle for liberty as the earlier and more successful struggle of I776" (Belin 259). While metaphor may certainly, at times, originate in an "impulse to escape from the world," it more often reflects a desire, even a need, to expand and revivify the world by offering new formulations for things newly seen, discovered, or created—that is, for new things.

On one hand, then, a transit from self to other, known to unknown, familiar and customary to foreign and novel. But this formulation is only part of the story. Although some of the terms I have been using—revelation, unfolding scene of instruction, vector, and so on (see above, pp. 19–22, for example)—imply a one-directional sequence, the act of knowing can also be conceived in a contrary way: not as a venturing into new territory—or as a venturing that is only a first step—but as a new inclusion of that territory as part of the self's familiar environment or *Lebenswelt.* What Max Black terms "an *interaction* view of metaphor" suggests that while the vehicle of the metaphor shapes our view of the tenor, the reverse is also true. "If to call a man a wolf is to put him in a special light," argues Black, "we must not forget that the metaphor makes the wolf seem more human than he otherwise would" (Black, "Metaphor" 285, 290). Not simply X = Y, then, but, as in a reversible chemical reaction, X ⇔Y. To adapt the language of a "replacement" view of metaphor, a metaphor replaces X not with Y alone but with X *and* Y. In Ricoeur's formulation, "The metaphor is not the vehicle alone, but the whole made up of the two halves" (Ricoeur 80). "The tenor does not remain unaltered, as if the vehicle were nothing but wrapping and decoration" (Ricoeur 81). Consequently, "the simultaneous presence of the tenor and vehicle and their interaction engender the metaphor" (Ricoeur 81). From this perspective, the processing of a metaphor involves a movement from self to other, but also, on the other hand, a complementary movement from other to self, vehicle to tenor: a kind of *introjection* of an initially foreign and external object or concept.

Otherness and Predication. Metaphor and the Uncanny

Walker Percy explores this play between tenor and vehicle, presence and otherness, partly by elaborating on a passage from Cassirer's *Language and Myth.* Percy recalls that while hunting with his father, brother, and a guide,

> we saw a wonderful bird. He flew as swift and straight as an arrow, then all of a sudden folded his wings and dropped like a stone into the woods. I asked what the bird was. The guide said it was a Blue Dollar Hawk. Later my father told me … it was really a Blue Darter Hawk. I can still remember my disappointment at the correction.
>
> *(Percy 79)*

This is one of the moments on which Percy builds his argument that the incorrect or metaphoric name for the bird, unlike the "correct" or conventional one, reveals a combination of power and mystery that conveys not the descriptive features of the hawk (blue, darting, and so on) but something of its very being. The correct phrase describes the bird. The incorrect one, precisely through its mistakenness ("Metaphor as Mistake"), gives us something new: the essential individuality or whatness of the bird.

"The next moment," says Percy, is "the most remarkable of all, because it can receive no explanation in the conventional sign theory of meaning":

> The boy, having perfectly perceived the flight of the hawk, now suffers a sort of disability, a tension, even a sense of imminence! He puts the peculiar question, *what is that bird?*, and puts it importunately. He is really anxious to know. But to know what? … Why does he want an answer at all? He has already apprehended the hawk in the vividest, most plenary way—a sight he will never forget as long as he lives. What more will he know by having the bird named? … We have come already to the heart of the question … For the situation of the boy in Alabama is very much the same sort of thing as what Cassirer calls the "mythico-religious Urphenomenon." Cassirer … emphasized the situation in which the primitive comes face to face with something which is both entirely new to him and strikingly distinctive, so distinctive that it might be said to have a *presence … And it is in the two ways in which this tensional encounter is resolved that the Urphenomenon is said to beget metaphor and myth.*
>
> *(Percy 84–5, my italics except for* "presence." *Percy seems to rely principally on pp. 17–18 in Cassirer, but other pertinent discussions appear on 28–33, 83–5, and 88–9)*

The first way is through the mysterious power "born of the sense of unformulated presence of the thing." This is the power of the phenomenon's *otherness* to the boy, or to the "primitive," or to whoever is having the experience. The second way is through the linguistic formulation of the experience: "the metaphor arises from the symbolic act in which the emotional cry of the beholder becomes the vehicle by which the thing is conceived, the name of the thing" (Percy 85). This is the power of the *self* to name the phenomenon, to make it one's own, to come to possess it. In William Melaney's words, such an encounter "bespeaks the unthinkable coalescence of a peculiar shock and the duality of metaphor." It is "both a sudden and unpredictable response to lived experience and a formation of new meaning" (Melaney 53, paraphrasing Jacques Rancière on Marcel Proust).

The doubleness of this experience resonates suggestively with the phenomenon of the uncanny, which in turn intersects profoundly with the concept of metaphor. What Percy calls "the sense of unformulated presence of the thing," for example, recalls Jacques Lacan's contention that "There is no cognitive dissonance here, we rather cross all possible cognition, to find ourselves in the field where we do not know how to distinguish bad and good, pleasure from displeasure. And this is the signal of anxiety: the signal of the Real, as irreducible to any signifier" (https://artandpopularculture.com/Uncanny#Lacan. NB: This passage appears, often but not always as punctuated here, in several places on the internet—for example, https://www.artandpopularculture.com/L'angoisse—but none offers a precise source. So I must add the obligatory "provenance uncertain"). Although she does not make this claim in *Powers of Horror*, one might even see a link between Empson's idea of "resistance to a false identity"—an identity threatening to undo the symbolic order—and Julia Kristeva's concept of "abjection": a need to expel from the self what is socially interdicted and must be separated or shed or "abjected." Compare Roland Barthes' conceptually parallel remark, in *S/Z*: "The ultimate horror is not death but that the classification of death and life should be broken off" (Barthes 107). Put simply, the indeterminacies of the uncanny deprive us of the definitions, names, clarities, distinctions associated with the Lacanian Symbolic and thus to some extent evoke the Real—that sphere of experiences without determinate conceptual or linguistic identity. Thus formulations like those noted immediately above: "unformulated presence," "unthinkable coalescence," and the like.

Whether the unfolding of the metaphoric process is understood as moving from tenor to vehicle or from vehicle to tenor, the interpreter (reader or hearer) is in two different relations to the object: a relation of largely unproblematic clarity, familiarity, and mastery, and a relation of obscurity, strangeness, uncertainty, and distress. These relations recall the two subject-positions marking the mechanism of the Freudian notion of the Uncanny, and of its predecessor, the "intellectual uncertainty" and "lack of orientation" of Ernst Jentsch's *On the Psychology of the Uncanny*. But to bring out the uncanny dimensions of metaphor, which is inescapably a linguistic and sociocultural and not just a purely individual phenomenon, we must shift the context from the individual psyche to the sphere of the symbolic order: the sphere, in Lacan's terms, of the social, the cultural, the conceptual, the symbolic, the linguistic, the rule-bound, and so on.

This portion of my argument attempts to develop two main assertions. The first is that metaphor and the uncanny are analogous structures. The second is that the unconscious in the individual psyche has a sociocultural counterpart in a kind of cultural reservoir both linguistic and conceptual. The first assertion claims that the twofold structure of the uncanny, in which the *heimlich* and the *unheimlich* fuse into a single tensional and self-contradictory relationship, is replayed or mirrored in the relationship of tenor and vehicle in metaphor. X is Y means that there is only one thing, *and* that there are two. That is, the *heimlich* tenor is both distinct from the *unheimlich* vehicle and identified with it, as the truth in metaphor is both distinct from its falsity and identified with it. This connection is implicitly suggested by the oxymoronic character of the language shared by Freud's description of the uncanny and Ricoeur's description of metaphor. For Freud, the uncanny is "in reality nothing new or foreign, but something familiar and old." It is "that class of the terrifying which leads back to something long known to us, once very familiar … nothing else than a hidden, familiar thing," or as the Standard Edition has it, something that is "secretly familiar." (See Standard Edition, vol. 17, p. 245: "It may be true that the uncanny [*unheimlich*] is something which is secretly familiar [*heimlich-heimisch*], which has undergone repression and then returned from it, and that everything that is uncanny fulfils this condition." Indeed, the very word "*heimlich* is not unambiguous … on the one hand, it means that which is familiar and congenial, and on the other, that which is kept out of sight.") In the end, in fact, the opposition between *heimlich* and *unheimlich* is impossible to sustain because the meaning of *heimlich* "develops towards an ambivalence, until it finally coincides with its opposite, *unheimlich. Unheimlich* is in some way or other a sub-species of *heimlich*" (Freud, "The 'Uncanny'" 13, 1–2, 4). New and old, terrifying and long known to us, foreign and familiar, secretly familiar, familiar and congenial but out of sight, both *heimlich* and *unheimlich* (the latter being finally a "sub-species" of the former)—the uncanny is inescapably self-contradictory, paradoxical, oxymoronic.

As is metaphor. For Ricoeur, following Beardsley, metaphor is similarly self-contradictory, and thus a cousin of oxymoron.

> Oxymoron is the simplest sort of meaningful self-contradiction (to live a living death). Within the domain of what is normally called metaphor, contradiction is more indirect … Let us say, then, that "whenever an attribution is indirectly self-contradictory, and the modifier has connotations that could be attributed to the subject, the attribution is a *metaphorical attribution*, or metaphor."
>
> *(Ricoeur 95. The internal quotation is from Beardsley,* Aesthetics *141)*

Ricoeur elaborates, focusing on

> the inescapably paradoxical character surrounding a metaphorical concept of truth. The paradox consists in the fact that there [NB: I have corrected Ricoeur's text from "there there" to "that there"] is no other way to do justice to the notion of metaphorical truth than to include the critical incision of the (literal) "is not" within the ontological vehemence of the (metaphorical) "is." In doing so, the thesis merely draws the most extreme consequence of the theory of tension.
>
> *(Ricoeur 255)*

That is, in asserting "X is Y," metaphor must—in effect—deal with Butler's objection that "Every thing is what it is, and not another thing." To do so, it endorses both assertion and objection by means of Ricoeur's claim that, in addition to the everyday "is" ("Donald is a devilish coprolite"), there is a second "is" that plunges us into the inescapable and self-contradictory duality of metaphoric assertion by meaning "is and is not" (Ricoeur 255). Whether or not it is necessary or even justifiable to posit such a second "is," Ricoeur's most insistent and essential contention is that what metaphor predicates of an object or abstraction or entity is inescapably self-contradictory, oxymoronic. And it is here, in the final string of phrases with which he distinguishes ordinary from metaphoric predication, that Ricoeur's language about metaphor most directly echoes Freud's language about the paradoxical and oxymoronic aspects of the uncanny.

> Literal application [of a predicate] is simply the one that has been endorsed by usage. This is why the question of truth is not restricted or peculiar. Only metaphorical application is peculiar: for extension in the application of a label or a schema must *satisfy opposed demands—it must be new but fitting, strange but evident, surprising but satisfying.*
>
> *(Ricoeur 236–7, my italics)*

Ricoeur's phrasing closely echoes Freud's formulation that the uncanny is, "in reality nothing new or foreign, but something familiar and old … that class of the terrifying which leads back to something long known to us," "secretly familiar."

In his compact and lucid study, David Punter also sees in metaphor a "dialectic of similarity and difference," though for me it is a dialectic without synthesis or transcendence—that is, an inescapably contestatory structure and movement. Thus when Punter argues further that this dialectic "might remind us of the collection of experiences and factors which we refer to under the heading 'the uncanny,'" I certainly agree, but his dividing the focus between similarity in some chapters and difference in others indicates, symbolically, a great distance between our conceptualizings of metaphor (Punter 87–8).

The structure of Freud's (and Jentsch's) uncanny maps onto the structure of metaphor in such a way that—to begin with, at least—conscious is to unconscious as tenor is to vehicle. "To begin with" because, as we have already begun to note, the question of which—tenor or vehicle—is the normative-conventional term and which the disruptive outlier does not always yield a simple answer, any more than does the question whether the terms can be separated. Assuredly, *tenor* and *vehicle* are in some sense rival terms, but as Coleridge reminds us, "Antagonist forces are necessarily of the **same** kind … *Inter res heterogeneas non datur oppositio*; that is, contraries cannot be opposites … Rivals (*rivales*) are those only who inhabit the opposite banks of the **same** stream" (Coleridge 26–7, my boldface of both instances of "same"). The complexity of this relation is evident, as we have seen, in Fielding's strategy in his *Modern Glossary*. For the *Glossary* to function as a satiric text, the older, conventional meanings of words must not be displaced but must carry over into the discursive sphere of the newer debased meanings, and it is the tension between them that generates Fielding's satire in this work.

Things are further problematized by Julian Jaynes's apparent reversal of the roles of tenor and vehicle. "In every metaphor," he writes, "there are at least two terms, the thing we are trying to express in words, the metaphrand, and the term produced to do so, the metaphier." These terms "are similar to what Richards (1936) called the tenor and the vehicle …" (Jaynes, "Consciousness" 132).

Again, "There are thus always two terms in a metaphor, the thing to be described, which I shall call the *metaphrand*, and the thing or relation used to elucidate it, which I shall call the *metaphier*. **A metaphor is always a known metaphier operating on a less known metaphrand**" (Jaynes, *Origin* 48–9, my boldface). By this last sentence, Jaynes is suggesting, I believe, that the metaphrand (tenor) is "less known" because—contrary to normative opinion—there is much to be revealed beneath its conventional surface, and that this revealing is accomplished by the metaphier (vehicle). So in "The governor is a fox," the vehicle or new term—fox—is something we are understood to know, but the governor, or tenor, is something we *thought* we knew but is shown to have been only incompletely known once the vehicle discloses the tenor's full vulpine meaning. As Jaynes's explanation suggests, it is easy to confuse these terms and operations—at least, to understand them in multiple ways (as in the somewhat uncertain anthropological exposition of Durham and Fernandez, 191–2).

The Psychoanalytic vs. the Sociocultural Uncanny

If metaphor and the uncanny are analogous structures, then the familiar or *heimlich* tenor of an individual (or an individual's) metaphor is in the sociocultural context inextricably tied to the sphere of correctness, custom, and usage. Likewise, the unfamiliar or wayward or *unheimlich* vehicle of a metaphor conceived as an individual utterance is tied to the individual psyche's unconscious. But the unconscious in the individual psyche or psychoanalytic sphere must have a sociocultural counterpart that is a kind of cultural reservoir both linguistic and conceptual. Unlike the individual unconscious, this reservoir is not a place to which things have been consigned (repressed) because they are unacceptable but a place from which things have not been liberated because they are *not yet* acceptable, or even recognized. Like a mythical golden age, but in reverse, this reservoir is not directly or presently available: historically, because it is located in the future as the golden age is located in the unreachable mythic past, and modally, because its status is mythical in the sense that its contents are latent or virtual rather than realized. The situation is the inverse of what René Girard's compelling book title terms *Des choses cachées depuis la fondation du monde* (derived from NASB, Matthew 13:35: "things hidden since the foundation of the world"). The reservoir I am speaking of harbors things hidden until the culture allows them to be made manifest. Until, that is, the uncanny reveals or "realizes" them—a dynamic that is caught in Freud's citation of Schelling: "'Unheimlich' is the name for everything that ought to have remained … hidden and secret *and has become visible*" (Freud, "The 'Uncanny'" 3–4, my emphasis; Schelling 649). The notion of such a "reservoir" reminds us, once more, that metaphor itself is made possible not just by individual persons and their discourse but also by its sociocultural context at any given moment. In a sense, the link between metaphor and the uncanny is itself based on an initial metaphoric transformation, from context of individual psyche to context of sociocultural norms and challenges to those norms.

A more concertedly historical—past-focused, even quasi-archaeological—version of this "reservoir" or stockpile, like that of Hans Blumenberg in *Paradigms for a Metaphorology* and other texts, is described by the translator of *Paradigms* in this way:

> The vicissitudes of metaphor—the replacement of one metaphor by another, or the accretions in meaning undergone by a single metaphor—are the subject of a new form of historiography that probes texts for evidence of the conceptually irrecoverable presuppositions on which they operate, the "*cultural subconscious to which they give involuntary expression.*"
>
> *(Robert Savage, in Blumenberg,* Paradigms *144, my italics)*

Savage elaborates on this mode of historiography: "I borrow the term 'cultural subconscious' from Rüdiger Zill, who describes metaphorology as '*the cultural-historical pendant to the psychoanalysis of the individual*'" (Zill 31, my emphasis). This is an economical and accurate characterization of Blumenberg's "archaeological" project. Yet "pendant" does not begin to suggest how much the singular features of what Zill terms the "cultural subconscious"—though its structure and mechanisms are analogous to those of the individual psyche—differ from the features of the individual model.

The antithesis between the tenor of a metaphor and the vehicle, as I have said, is parallel to the opposition between the *heimlich* and the *unheimlich*, as well as between the conscious and the unconscious. The tenor-*heimlich*-individual ego representative takes the form of all those linguistic-conceptual elements that are conventional or culturally sanctioned—elements that are aligned with established usage and custom. In contrast, the *sociocultural counterparts* to the individual psyche, the unconscious, and the *unheimlich*, take the form of the sociocultural sphere as a whole, its reservoir or cache, and its contents that are unrealized rather than repressed. What is outside the sphere of custom and usage, unknown and unnumbered in that cultural cache that corresponds to the individual unconscious, is exactly the opposite of what Alexander Pope describes as "True Wit" in *An Essay on Criticism* (lines 297–300):

True wit is nature to advantage dress'd,
What oft was thought, but ne'er so well express'd,
Something, whose truth convinc'd at sight we find,
That gives us back the image of our mind.

This is the discourse of the known ("nature," in the eighteenth-century sense) and familiar ("What oft was thought"), transformed only in that the poet has "dress'd" it "to advantage," thus confining the singularity ("ne'er") of the utterance/thought not to its meaning but to its being "so well express'd." To the extent that aphoristic discourse like Pope's seems to articulate a timeless or previously formulated truth, it presents itself as, so to speak, "already read" and thus requires only to be re-cognized. The text expresses "Something, whose truth convinc'd at sight we find,/That gives us back the image of our mind." Such a text is scarcely "other" at all, and Pope's lines appropriately fuse truth and reader into a single entity, partly through the two senses of "convince": the modern sense, but also the older one, "to demonstrate conclusively" (see *OED*, s.v. "convince," II.6.7.8). This syntactic strategy portrays the text as giving us something that we already know—and are. The text's assertions are "convinced," and so are we.

Such discourse is "proper" in more than one sense. In the first place, it is correct, culturally sanctioned, conventional, governed by "usage"—*echt heimlich.* In the second, it is proper in the sense derived from French *propre*: [one's] own, belonging to. That is, the signifier is so regularly attached to the signified (object/concept/person) that it seems to "belong" to it—even, at times, to be its "natural" rather than its conventional name. In terms of metaphor, it is the discourse of the tenor. "The uncanny," as Nicholas Royle helpfully says,

> is a crisis of the proper: it entails a critical disturbance of what is proper … a disturbance of the very idea of personal or private property including the properness of proper names, one's so-called 'own' name, but also the proper names of others, of places, institutions and events.
>
> *(Royle 1)*

The discourse of the vehicle is very different. If the discourse of the tenor is, in a sense, that of the ego as governed by the superego—in sociocultural terms, the community as regulated by convention and usage—the discourse of the vehicle is that of a reservoir of linguistic-conceptual virtuality, unlimited and unrestrained, generated by the fertility of what we could figuratively term a cultural id or unconscious. This reservoir contains everything that might conceivably (but also inconceivably!) serve as the vehicle of a metaphor—however fresh, startling, inappropriate, surreal, or impossible—but has not yet become so. These potential metaphoric vehicles are not—or not yet—culturally approved or adopted. They are strange, *unheimlich*, improper in both senses mentioned above: unsuitable or incorrect, and "other" to the discourse of the sociocultural ego—the latter describable as the existent word hoard disciplined by usage. The clash between elements of this reservoir and elements of conventional usage is what produces the sociocultural and linguistic-conceptual counterpart of the uncanny.

Freud summarizes the two sources of the uncanny (as experienced by the individual psyche) in this way: "An uncanny experience occurs either when repressed infantile complexes have been revived by some impression, or when the primitive beliefs we have surmounted seem once more to be confirmed" (Freud, "The 'Uncanny'" 17). For Mark Windsor, the second theory—"the apparent confirmation of 'surmounted primitive beliefs'"—is "the one that faces fewer serious objections and carries greater explanatory power in respect to the uncanny" (Windsor 35). Those primitive beliefs include a "narcissistic over-estimation of subjective mental processes" (such as the ability to bring about events merely by thinking or wishing them), along with a belief that the world is "peopled with the spirits of human beings," that the dead may survive as spirits, and that the material world—in particular, the natural world—is not merely inert or organic but populated by animistic spirits (Freud, "The 'Uncanny'" 12–13). In such a world, what are to most people natural objects, places, landscapes, and creatures are inhabited by a spiritual essence—are animated and alive much as humans are. Fairies, demons, dryads, hamadryads, *genii loci*, spirits of earth or sky or water, and other beings populate this world and provide it with a range of phenomena unknown to merely naturalistic thinkers. (Here I am still paraphrasing a well-known passage from Freud, 12–13.) Once we move from the realm of the individual psyche to that of the sociocultural or linguistic-conceptual, however, such animistic figures are replaced by the boundless and novel contents of the cultural reservoir that we are exploring.

From a *modern* critical perspective, that is, what all the instances of animistic beings share, in addition to their animism, is that they are tokens of an enlarged conception of reality: a world with more things and beings—and kinds of thing and being—than we find in our ordinary or everyday or naturalistic world. In terms of the structure of metaphor, what Freud describes as the (modern) capacity of humans to view seemingly animistic phenomena critically aligns with the tenor, and thus with its operation under the aegis of the conventional, the known, the culturally sanctioned and familiar. The vehicle, on the other hand, or the cache of vehicles from which individual vehicles are drawn, replaces the primitive extra-worldly array of animistic creatures and phenomena—"the primitive beliefs we have surmounted [and that] seem once more to be confirmed," in Freud's words—with the *modern* extra-worldly: that is, with the potential, virtual, novel, not-yet-realized array of possible predicates in the metaphoric assertion that X is Y. Recall Ricoeur's distinction, cited earlier:

> Literal application [of a predicate] is simply the one that has been endorsed by usage. This is why the question of truth is not restricted or peculiar. *Only metaphorical application is peculiar: for extension in the application of a label or a schema must satisfy opposed demands—it must be new but fitting, strange but evident, surprising but satisfying.*
>
> (*Ricoeur 236–7, my italics*)

If there is a link in Freud's account, then, between the revived or confirmed "primitive beliefs" and the reemergence of the supernatural, there is another link between the vehicle of a given metaphor and the now disclosed but heretofore hidden dimensions of the world it makes manifest. One need not posit a primitive stage of civilization in which the world was more abundantly populated with magical, supernatural things and beings than it is now. All that is required is the common experience or sensation that the world is or may be different from, especially richer or more abundant than, our conventional experience of it. As Bernard Malamud cheerfully says, "I love metaphor. It provides two loaves where there seems to be one" (Nordquist n. pag.). Malamud was anticipated by Samuel Johnson, who remarked to James Boswell in September 1777: "Sir, as to metaphorical expression, that is a great excellence in style, when it is used with propriety, for it gives you two ideas for one;—conveys the meaning more luminously, and generally with a perception of delight" (Boswell 855).

This sequence of reasoning has taken us from the individual unconscious and its repressed material to its sociocultural counterpart: to the idea of a hidden and unconventional vision of the world and to the movement within a metaphor from the tenor, which expresses the conventional understanding of the world, to the vehicle, which discloses a new understanding. The latter is inevitably, at first, "wondrous strange," as Horatio says in *Hamlet*. In reply, Hamlet interestingly affirms the reality of this strangeness—"There are more things in heaven and earth, Horatio,/Than are dreamt of in your philosophy"—but not before urging that Horatio treat the "strange" as a traveling "stranger," and "give it welcome" (I.v.185–6. Cf. KJV, Hebrews 13:2: "Be not forgetful to entertain strangers: for thereby some have entertained angels unawares"). That urging adumbrates the embrace of the vehicle as a revision or replacement of the tenor—a replacement that offers new multiplicity and abundance, and indeed newness—or novelty—as such.

8

NOVELTY AND THE END STATE OF METAPHOR

Uncanny Doubling

The Two Sides of Novelty

To summarize: the tenor-*heimlich*-individual ego representative takes the form of all those linguistic-conceptual elements that are conventional or culturally sanctioned—elements aligned with established usage. The vehicle-*unheimlich*-sociocultural representative offers the promise of the surprising, the unknown, the daring and expansive: in short, the novel. The valorization of novelty dates to some of the earliest writings on metaphor. For Aristotle, "To learn easily is naturally pleasant to all people," and "metaphor most brings about learning … A simile is less pleasing because longer," and because—unlike metaphor—"it does not say that this is that, nor does [the listener's] mind seek to understand this" (*Aristotle on Rhetoric* 218). Without metaphor, *this* remains *this* and cannot attain to the novelty of *that*.

In addition to the attestations of Black, Cassirer, Nowottny, and others (see Chapter 5), more recent writers on figurative language also insist on the operations of metaphor as the discovery or creation of new meanings and definitions. Dennis Potter, for example, writes of the "flickering into life of the world behind the world which, of course, is what all metaphors" are about (Nordquist n. pag.). Potter's language economically points to the sense of hidden abundance often intimated by figurative language and by art more generally. I suggest that it is not so much a matter of "before" and "behind" as of the actual and the virtual—the latter being the potential world or worlds that might be realized from the latent meanings constituting the cultural reserve of the linguistic-conceptual. And Jaynes, countering the claim that "metaphor is a mere comparison and cannot make new entities," insists that the "grand and vigorous function of metaphor is the generation of new language as it is needed, as human culture becomes more and more complex."

DOI: 10.4324/9781003560050-8

Metaphors not only increase our perception and understanding of the world but "literally create new objects. Indeed, language is an organ of perception, not simply a means of communication." Here, Jaynes closely echoes Cassirer: "Thus the special symbolic forms are not imitations, but *organs* of reality, since it is solely by their agency that anything real becomes an object for intellectual apprehension, and as such is made visible to us" (Jaynes, "Consciousness" 132, 7; Jaynes, *Origin* 49, 50; Cassirer 8, my italics). In the language of the present study, Jaynes's "new objects" are conceived not so much as products of the individual imagination as revelations from or glimpses into a vast sociocultural "space": the linguistic and conceptual counterpart to the psychic unconscious that I have termed a reservoir, cache, or limitless stockpile of latent metaphoric vehicles.

The association of metaphor with newness and discovery typically generates an appreciation of boldness and invention: sometimes of a figure of speech poetically fresh and surprising, like Yeats's "An aged man is but a paltry thing,/A tattered coat upon a stick ..." (W. B. Yeats, "Sailing to Byzantium" 9–10); sometimes of utterances more vatic and apocalyptic, like this declamation of Blake's: "What it will be Questiond, When the Sun rises do you not see a round Disk of fire somewhat like a Guinea O no no I see an Innumerable company of the Heavenly host crying Holy Holy Holy is the Lord God Almighty" (Blake 565–6).

But when we look at the obverse of this familiar celebration of novelty and expanded vision—of the ability of metaphors to increase our perceived reality—we approach the dark side of the uncanny more closely. For the creation of each new object by means of metaphoric transformation is also, and unavoidably, the alteration, or dimming, or crossing out of the original object. As soon as the speaker of Shelley's best-known ode, for example, utters its opening phrase, "O wild West Wind, thou breath of Autumn's being," he inaugurates a process of redefinition and replacement in which tenor and vehicle, abetted by the personification and apostrophe that render the West Wind addressable, vie for primacy in a now contestatory definitional space (see Goodman, *Languages of Art* 69, discussed on pp. 9, 22, above). On the one hand, the familiar tenor, the West Wind. On the other, the surprising and novel vehicle, the "breath of Autumn's being." In an admittedly fanciful allegorization of the poem as a one-sided conversation not between poet and West Wind but between tenor and vehicle, one might imagine the speaker's desire to have the wind-spirit become his spirit, even to have it commandeer his selfhood ("Be thou me, impetuous one!"—that is, not "Be or become me!" but "Replace my being with yours!"), as the plangent desire of the tenor firmly embedded in conventional language—and aware of its imminent erasure—to be entirely swallowed up by the visionary reality of the vehicle. The poem expresses this desire, but it does not register its fulfillment. The wind-spirit is asked both to receive the speaker's utterance—"hear, oh hear!"—and (via the pun) to be present to him as well: *here, oh here!* But the silence of the spirit and the distance inferred from the very expression of the longing for presentness leave his prayer unfulfilled.

The End State of Metaphor

Indeed, to continue the analogy between Shelley's ode and the dynamics of metaphor, that prayer could be answered and fulfilled only at the hypothetical end of the metaphoric process, when the phrase-concept "wild West Wind" has vanished and the breath of Autumn's being has shed its figurative status and become the new—literal—tenor. At any given moment, a particular metaphor may exist at one or another point in this process. The vehicle may be gently marginal or penumbral to a still largely dominant tenor. It may exist in a balance where meaning wavers uncertainly between tenor and vehicle. Or the vehicle may—at least theoretically—entirely subsume or replace the tenor, the metaphoric process thereby reaching an "ideal" completion. "Words become metaphors for other things," as William Gass says, "then slowly disappear into the new image" (Nordquist n. pag.). At such moments, of course, the metaphor itself ceases to exist and is knowable only by an inference or reconstruction from a now thoroughly literal phrase or concept: a reconstruction, in Blumenberg's words, "that probes texts for evidence of the conceptually irrecoverable presuppositions on which they operate" (Savage, "Translator's Afterword," in Blumenberg, *Paradigms* 144). Metaphor cannot express but can only gesture toward that moment.

Perhaps the closest we can come to observing this metaphoric end state is in a figure of speech like Pascal's famous redefinition of "man," at the beginning of one of his best-known *Pensées* (Léon Brunschvicg numbering, 347): "L'homme n'est qu'un roseau, le plus faible de la nature; mais c'est un roseau pensant" [Man is but a reed, the most feeble thing in nature; but it is a thinking reed].

"L'homme n'est qu'un roseau" is usually and reasonably translated as "Man is nothing but a reed." But Pascal did not in fact write "L'homme n'est **rien d'autre** qu'un roseau." Literally, the French says "Man is **not but** a reed." The usual translation softens Pascal's meaning by permitting a residual thinghood insofar as the "rien" ("nothing") in "rien d'autre" serves as a kind of placeholder for the shadowy "something" that it excludes. The literal makes stronger and clearer that there is a negation, an annihilation of *man*, as if to say, "The concept *man* exists no longer and henceforth will only appear and be recognized *as a reed*." This is the language not just of revision or redefinition, but of negation or—in psychoanalytic language—of repression. For the sign "man" to exist or appear from this point on, it will need to be de-repressed, dragged from the unconscious into the sphere of the conscious—again, like the uncanny in Schelling's definition: "everything that ought to have remained … hidden and secret and has become visible," or knowable. By placing the man that is no longer and the reed that has replaced him in the same sentence, Pascal creates a tension that could rightly be called uncanny, because the sentence names what it affirms does not exist. A modern and more Derridean

Pascal might have placed the word *sous rature* (under erasure), thus: "~~L'homme~~ n'est qu'un roseau." But the expedient of erasure is not required since the syntax of the sentence as written creates a tension by at once referring to the concept and announcing its annihilation. This is the uncanny as shrewdly defined by Katherine Withy in her valuable *Heidegger on Being Uncanny*: "an irresolvable uncertainty about the applicability of the very categories that we use"—in this case, the categories of existence and nonexistence (Withy 18; and see Taylor Carman's subtle and appreciative review of Withy in *European Journal of Philosophy*).

Finally, the "completion" of the metaphorical process that Pascal's figure approaches may recall my earlier discussion in which process and temporality link the reader's gradual comprehension of a metaphor, the unfolding syntax of English sentences, the educative and even revelatory dimensions of this quasi-narrative unfolding, and more (see above, pp. 18–21). All rest on the fact that the simplest statement of an identity, like "X is Y," names an atemporal relationship (identity) but does so in an inescapably temporal mode because X precedes Y in the actual utterance (see Chapter 2). Here is what *Etymonline* offers under "metaphor":

> "figure of speech by which a characteristic of one object is assigned to another, different but resembling it or analogous to it; comparison by transference of a descriptive word or phrase," late 15c., *methaphoris* (plural), from French *metaphore* (Old French *metafore*, 13c.) and directly from Latin *metaphora*, [b] **from Greek *metaphora* "a transfer," especially of the sense of one word to a different word, literally "a carrying over," from *metapherein* "to transfer, carry over; change, alter; to use a word in a strange sense," from *meta* "over, across" (see** meta-**) + *pherein* to carry, bear."**
>
> *(https://www.etymonline.com, s.v. "metaphor." Accessed 12 January 2020. Boldface mine.)*

(For a particularly rich account of links between metaphor and the notion of a carrying-over, see Zanker, especially chapter 8, "The Classical Metaphors for Metaphor," and more especially, chapter 8, section I, "The Spatial Metaphor of *μεταφορά* and *translatio*.")

The idea of metaphor as a movement or passage or journey is deeply embedded in the word's history.

Uncanny Doubling

But that process or passage takes on a different character when seen in its relation to the uncanny. Metaphor entails the repeated double-take of two conflicting versions of the "same" object, a double-take that is a first and a second looking but also a restless movement between them: at once an inchoate uncertainty and an unstable double-vision, somewhat like those that define the territory of the uncanny. Here, metaphor is not just a static juxtaposition and doubling of two terms, tenor and vehicle, but also something of an under-defined and perilous passage from one to the other, recalling, again, Lacan's description of the uncanny as a place where we "find ourselves in the field where we do not know how to distinguish bad and good, pleasure from displeasure. And this is the signal of anxiety: the signal of the Real, as irreducible to any signifier" (see p. 58 above). Put simply, the indeterminacies of the uncanny deprive us of the definitions, names, clarities, and distinctions associated with the Lacanian Symbolic and thus to some extent evoke the Real—the absence of determinate conceptual or linguistic outlines or identities.

A further dimension of this doubling process concerns the relation of the tenor not to the vehicle but to itself. This is a doubling between the tenor in its full semantic and ontological being and the tenor as it begins to be rendered fragile or indistinct by the competing energy of the vehicle. If the relation of sameness and difference between tenor and vehicle is uncanny, so is that between the pre-metaphoric tenor, linguistically and culturally stable, and the tenor as it enters into the structure of the metaphor. The doubling of tenor by vehicle, that is, inaugurates the disclosure and development of the tenor (T) as doubled by its own ghostly Doppelgänger or proleptic death mask (T^1). Further, the latter situation is a harbinger of the fragility of any and all customary understandings of things. After this first blow, all phrases, signs, and understandings under the aegis of conventionality and usage are rendered mortal. The situation recalls Freud's observation that "the familiar can become uncanny and frightening" (Freud, "The 'Uncanny'" 2), and is analogous to the effect of the grotesque in Wolfgang Kayser's account:

> The grotesque is a structure. Its nature could be summed up in a phrase that has repeatedly suggested itself to us: THE GROTESQUE IS THE ESTRANGED WORLD … We are so strongly affected and terrified because it is our world which ceases to be reliable, and we feel that we would be unable to live in this changed world. The grotesque … presupposes that the categories which apply to our world view become inapplicable.
>
> *(Kayser 184–5. Cf. Withy's remark*—Heidegger *18—that the uncanny entails "an irresolvable uncertainty about the applicability of the very categories that we use.")*

Such instances of doubling, involving as they do sameness and difference simultaneously, figure prominently in Slavoj Žižek's discussion of the double image of America in Hitchcock's *Psycho*, an image *divided between day and night*, "the hysteria of everyday capitalist life" and its "psychotic reverse: the nightmarish world of pathological crime." "The relationship between these two worlds," says Žižek, in a formulation that bears helpfully on the topic of metaphor and the uncanny, "eludes the simple oppositions of surface and depth, reality and fantasy, and so on—the only topology that suits it is that of the two surfaces of the Moebius band: if we progress far enough on one surface, all of a sudden we find ourselves on its reverse" (Žižek 227). I have called metaphor an "under-defined and perilous passage" between tenor and vehicle. Something similar can be said of movement along the Möbius strip which—among other oddities—creates a kind of cognitive dissonance between the senses of touch and sight. Holding a paper Möbius strip between two fingers, we distinctly feel the two sides of the paper. But when we turn from the tactile to the "ocular" proof, we discover that our fingers really touch only one side though at two different points. Lacan makes the point in a different way:

> If the insect that wanders along the surface of the Möbius strip [as in M. C. Escher's "Möbius Strip II, 1963"] forms a representation of the fact that it is a surface, he can believe from one moment to the next that there is another face that he hasn't explored, the face that is always on the back of the face along which he is walking. He can believe in this other side, even though there isn't one … Without knowing it, he is exploring the only face that there is, and yet, from one moment to the next, it does indeed have a back.
>
> *(Lacan, 136)*

Similarly, tenor and vehicle, in the abstract, are distinct entities, but at the same time, as the metaphor's copula (explicit or tacit) insists, they are one. "Nature is a temple."

If an image like the Möbius strip shows us the intimacy that can coexist with difference, it may simultaneously minimize the conflict that intimacy itself can generate—conflict that the vocabulary of doubling clearly implies. John Berryman dramatically compresses this drama of doubling in the opening line of "The Poet's Final Instructions," which includes his coinage "suisired." The word evokes "suicide," of course, but also suggests—*via* its Latin roots—a "siring" or fathering or begetting of oneself ("sui"). Such an act implies doubling of two kinds. On the one hand, to father oneself is to engage in a profoundly narcissistic act, sidestepping the need for a sexual or parental counterpart. As Freud says, following Otto Rank, "the 'double' was originally an insurance against destruction of the ego," a kind of spare or backup self rather than a "partner." On the other hand, the notion of "doubling as a preservation against extinction" takes a different form once the stage of primary narcissism has been outgrown: "From having been an assurance of immortality," the double becomes "the ghastly harbinger of death" (Freud, "The 'Uncanny'" 9). The intimacy of narcissistic identification issues in—is just the other side of—the ultimate self-alienating conflict that is suicide. Both meanings unite and contend in a single word. (I briefly discuss this word, "suisired," and its connections with *Paradise Lost*, V. 853–61, in Bogel, *New Formalist Criticism* 162–3.)

The uncanniness arises not from—or not so much from—the repeated or doubled element as from the conflictual mechanism of doubling itself. In Neil Hertz's formulation,

> The feeling of the uncanny would seem to be generated by being reminded of the repetition compulsion, not by being reminded of whatever it is that is repeated. The becoming aware of the process is felt as eerie, not the becoming aware of some particular item in the unconscious, once familiar, then repressed, now coming back into consciousness.

Hertz invokes Freud's *Beyond the Pleasure Principle* in support of this contention:

> "It may be presumed that when people unfamiliar with analysis feel an obscure fear—a dread of rousing something that, so they feel, is better left sleeping—what they are afraid of is the emergence of this compulsion with its hint of possession by some daemonic power."
>
> *(Freud, "Beyond,"* Standard Edition *18:36; Hertz 101–2)*

Thus, when an analysand during a psychoanalytic session casually mentions his brother, Abel, and simultaneously feels the *frisson* of his repressed image of the brother whose death he has wished for numerous times, what is important is less that there are two *Abels* than that there are *two* Abels. "It is," in Hertz's words again, "the emergence of the compulsion that they fear, as much as the reappearance of a particular fear or desire" (Hertz 102).

In a still more agonistic form, one capable of disrupting entire social groups as well as individual psyches, this mechanism reappears as René Girard's concept of "monstrous doubling," or "monstrous duality"—"the most disquieting and grotesque form [of "unity and reciprocity"] imaginable" (Girard, *Violence and the Sacred* 160). For Girard, desire is mimetic; we learn to desire an object through emulation of another's desire for it. But this imitative desire inescapably produces rivalry, and rivalry is a kind of classificatory breakdown insofar as the distinction between separate individuals is eroded—at least threatened—by the effort of both to claim or occupy the same position. In its expanded, socio-cultural form, this breakdown threatens to produce symmetrical violence such as we find in feuds, violence that extends the original structure of doubling or rivalry since all members of a particular group are potentially substitutable for all others. In a time of active feuding, any Hatfield or McCoy will do, not just the particular one—if there ever was one—who inaugurated the conflict. As a result, such violence is potentially endless. One faction attacks the other, the second retaliates; the first retaliates against the retaliation, and so on. "Vengeance," as Girard says, "is an interminable, infinitely repetitive process" (Girard 14. This paragraph borrows several lines from a discussion of doubling and satire in Bogel, *The Difference Satire Makes* 44).

Metaphor, doubling, the relation of the tenor to the vehicle, and of the tenor to itself—of T to V, and of T to T^1— Žižek's Möbius strip, the repetition compulsion and the repressed material it "disinters"—all of these conform to a single pattern or mechanism. Katherine Withy's discussion of Jentsch, in her *Heidegger on Being Uncanny*, helpfully clarifies what the mechanism of the uncanny is and is not:

> The uncertainty associated with the uncanny affect is not a temporary confusion about how to categorize an object (tree or snake?) but *an irresolvable uncertainty about the applicability of the very categories that we use* ... [The] tree/snake is either animate or inanimate rather than both and neither. To experience the uncanny affect, the traveler would have to have cause to wonder whether the entity is in fact a snake-tree … [S]imple mistakes about whether … [a] hand is prosthetic or not will not involve an uncanny affect. *Those objects that do reliably produce an uncanny affect are those that (seem to) span the distinction between animate and inanimate, like zombies and extremely lifelike robots.* So [Ernst] Jentsch's uncanniness of the unfamiliar, as illustrated in the tree/snake example, fails to capture the uncanny feeling because it involves a resolvable uncertainty, the locus of which is the entity itself rather than the categories in terms of which we make sense of it. *The unfamiliar is not itself uncanny but merely waiting to be made familiar … [W]hat must be added is that the unfamiliar thing be radically anomalous, in the sense that it calls the jointing of our 'ideational sphere' into question.*
>
> *(Withy 18, my italics)*

Despite her criticism in this passage, Withy hews more closely to Jentsch's essay on the uncanny than Freud's dismissive account does, patiently unpacking and extending Jentsch's emphasis on intellectual uncertainty and disorientation (compare Morlock's critique of Freud on Jentsch). She valuably reminds us that the uncertainty and shock of uncanny repetition arise not simply from two things or events, or from a thing whose identity is as yet uncertainly determined, but from uncertainty about one thing that equally seems to be two and therefore "destabilizes the realm of the familiar" (Withy 216). Adam Bresnick lucidly extends this instability to the self or subject experiencing the uncanny:

> The subject … palpably perceives the fact of his being inhabited by the constitutively foreign psychic agency of the unconscious. *The uncanny thus would not merely be something a given subject experiences, but the experience that momentarily undoes the factitious monological unity of the ego … It is in this fissuring of the subject, rather than in the specific content of the memory that occasions it, that Freud locates the disquieting affect of the uncanny.*
>
> *(Bresnick 117, my emphasis)*

In connection with Withy's use of Jentsch, I should note that I have not explored Freud's analysis of Hoffman's *The Sandman* in "The 'Uncanny,'" in part because its account of the story insists so exclusively on the motif of eyes and the castration-fear associated with the Oedipal complex; because it is so dismissive of Jentsch's contribution (and therefore trivializes the self-evidently central role of the doll-woman Olimpia); and because my focus is principally on the link between the uncanny and *metaphor*).

Intergalactic Excursus: Doubling, Metaphor, and *Star Trek*

Withy's teasing out of the uncertainty created by a single object that also seems to be two objects and thus "destabilizes the realm of the familiar"—along with Bresnick's understanding of the uncanny as an experience "that momentarily undoes the factitious monological unity of the ego"—foregrounds the uncertainty about boundaries that follows from metaphor's founding identity as a phenomenon at once true and false (Withy 216; Bresnick 117). The boundary between tenor and vehicle is only one locus of such uncertainty and uncanniness, but it is an essential one, capable of great variation and serving many different thematic ends.

In "Darmok," a 1991 episode of *Star Trek: The Next Generation*, for example, set in the twenty-fourth century, the crew of the *Enterprise* is unable to establish meaningful communication with the crew of a Tamarian ship. The Tamarians seem to speak obscurely and obliquely in what the crew decides are metaphors. More precisely, it gradually becomes clear that they communicate via brief allusions to their history and mythology in order to convey thoughts and intentions, ideas about action and attitude, and precedents for behavior.

For instance, Captain Picard and the crew are puzzled by such phrases as "Darmok and Jalad at Tanagra," "Temba, his arms wide," "The beast at Tanagra," and "Kiazi's children, their faces wet." Gradually realizing that these phrases are citations or invocations of, or allusions to, persons, places, and events drawn from Tamarian history, myth, and literature, Picard has a "Eureka" moment: "That's how you communicate, isn't it? By citing example. *By metaphor!*" Explaining the Tamarians' language further, crew member Deanna Troi tells Beverly Crusher that "It's as if I were to say to you, 'Juliet on her balcony,'" to which Crusher immediately responds, "An image of romance." "Exactly," says Troi. Narrative B is understood by being juxtaposed—even identified—with (prior) Narrative A.

So historical or mythico-literary events that are alluded to serve as vehicles illuminating a present situation that functions as the tenor of what one could call a narrative metaphor. Not just individual persons, things, and places but entire narrative segments can constitute the vehicle of these metaphors. This situation is similar to the way a heroic narrative—and perhaps the heroic mode as such—is juxtaposed with an everyday narrative and the ethos of the mundane in a mock-heroic text like Alexander Pope's *The Rape of the Lock*. In a kind of double-exposure or stereoscopic vision (see Chapter 4 above), episodes of Homeric or

Vergilian epic share the story with trivial activities of courtly society such as gossip, tea-drinking, and flirtation. In the case of the Tamarian metaphors we encounter in this episode, of course, the ironic effect we associate with mock-heroic does not appear, but the two levels of discourse do.

The Tamarians' discourse is not simply a management of metaphoric doubleness; their metaphoric juxtapositions powerfully emphasize closeness and identification and correspondingly minimize distance and difference. The metaphoric "is," for the Tamarians, is far stronger than the metaphoric "is not" with which we Terrestrials are familiar. (On Ricoeur and metaphor's "is not," see above, pp. 59–60.) Moreover, the reason for this particular inflection of metaphoric structure is more than linguistic, and powerfully thematic. At one point, the android Lieutenant Commander, Data, explains that "The Tamarian ego structure does not seem to allow what we normally think of as self-identity. Their ability to abstract is highly unusual." The Tamarians' attenuated (in human—or android—eyes) sense of self-identity means that they see humanoid entities as more *permeable* than do humans: more same than different, less jealously protective of isolated identity-hood. "My house is your house," but even "The dwellers in my house *are you*." That is why the Tamarian captain, Dathon, finds Picard's inability to comprehend the Tamarian language so frustrating: Picard is failing not simply to understand an analogue to their present situation but to understand a metaphoric vehicle that—almost without qualification—*is* their present situation.

It is as though the Tamarians want to purge metaphor of even the possibility of being understood on the model of simile, want to insist as much as possible on identification and not comparison, and do so by sharply limiting the role of difference in the structure of their metaphors. Not to comprehend that Darmok and Jalal in some sense *are* Picard and Dathon is a failure not simply to grasp an analogy but to understand Picard and Dathon at all, as well as a failure to recognize the literally unearthly uncanniness of their near identification.

It becomes inescapably clear, then, that the story is about the difference between two languages but also between two races or life forms, human and non-human. To discover the true relationship between tenor and vehicle of a Tamarian metaphor is also to discover the true relationship between Picard and Dathon: a relationship that at last succeeds in powerfully subordinating difference and separation to commonality and union. The episode is about language, but also about two species discovering their fundamental sameness and compatibility. It offers a dream of communication across a linguistic void and also a dream of creaturely connection across a desert of individualism. It is perhaps no accident that "Darmok" spelled backwards is "komrad."

9

THE UNCANNY

Psychoanalytic and Metaphoric

The uncanny shock of the return of the repressed must be distinguished from the shock produced by the "irresolvable uncertainty" of metaphor's uncanny. One way to begin is to ask what—in the metaphoric uncanny—stands in for the psychoanalytic uncanny's *Angst* arising from the return of the repressed: what Freud terms "all that is terrible," "all that arouses dread and creeping horror" (Freud, "'The 'Uncanny'" 1). For one thing, the metaphoric uncanny may produce a narrative, one strand of which turns into a "positive" story: if the tenor is threatened, eroded, and more or less undone by the vehicle, the narrative may nonetheless move toward the replacement of the former by the latter and thus toward an enlargement and even a reconfiguring—major or minor—of the conventional world: its language, concepts, and internal relationships. Pertinent here is T. S. Eliot's well-known literary-historical argument in "Tradition and the Individual Talent" that

> The existing order is complete before the new work arrives; for order to persist after the supervention of novelty, the *whole* existing order must be, if ever so slightly, altered; and so the relations, proportions, values of each work of art toward the whole are readjusted; and this is conformity between the old and the new.

Eliot concludes by asserting that it is not "preposterous that the past should be altered by the present as much as the present is directed by the past" (Eliot, "Tradition and the Individual Talent" 38–9). What begins as a "supervention of novelty" upon the existing order ends as an organic element of an order that has altered however slightly to accommodate that novelty.

DOI: 10.4324/9781003560050-9

Along with the "positive" narrative, however, there are anxieties and dreads and losses peculiar to the metaphoric uncanny. For one thing, since it alters what is known and how it is known, and what things and sorts of things do and do not exist, the metaphoric uncanny is a matter of affect but also of epistemological and ontological rearrangement or (in Eliot's vocabulary) readjustment. In addition, the "shock" of the metaphoric uncanny differs in character from that of the psychoanalytic uncanny. Schelling, we recall again, remarks that "'Unheimlich' is the name for everything that ought to have remained … hidden and secret and has become visible" (Freud, "The 'Uncanny'" 3–4). But the movement from hidden and secret to visible and known, as Freud notices, is an incomplete description. "Something has to be added to what is novel and unfamiliar to make it uncanny" (Freud, "The 'Uncanny'" 2). What is first hidden and then visible is also—having been "transformed by repression into morbid anxiety"—marked by something like danger, or shame, or aggression, or desire, or fear, or guilt, or the stigma of taboo, or several of these (Freud, "The 'Uncanny'" 13). That is why the moment when a boy inadvertently reveals to his mother that the rest of the family is secretly preparing a surprise birthday party for her is not an uncanny moment, even though the party had been hidden and secret and has now become revealed and known.

The shock of the metaphoric uncanny of course differs profoundly from the experience of, say, a soldier who had endured horrific battlefield terror on a day that happened to be his birthday and then, on a later birthday, is seized by or hurled into a traumatic reliving or de-repressing of the battlefield horrors he had consigned to psychic oblivion. (On Freud, combat, and war neuroses, see Cathy Caruth, *Unclaimed Experience: Trauma, Narrative, and History.*) The two kinds of shock are different for several reasons. First, of course, because the metaphoric uncanny is milder and usually less traumatic; it does not entail mortal fear, the possibility of one's own literal death, the spectacle of others killing and dying, and comparable horrors. Second, in the case of metaphor, the anxiety derives not simply from an instance of sexuality or aggression or some other unacceptable and therefore repressed individual thought or wish, but from the irruption into the conventional vision of experience of a new, heretofore hidden, vision of how and what the world is. Third, they differ because in the case of metaphor, the shock is not simply personal but socio-cultural as well: a displacement of the culturally conventional and usage-sanctioned concept/word/thing by an intrusion into that known world—an intrusion that may also efface certain elements of the familiar world as they are pushed off the stage by a new and formerly hidden element that is at once a death and a rebirth, an annihilation of some of the conventional world and an enlargement of it.

The Individual Unconscious and the Vehicle's Cultural Reservoir

Moreover, the psychoanalytic and the metaphoric uncanny differ with respect to the mechanisms of repression and the return of the repressed. Here is Withy's subtle revision of those Freudian mechanisms:

> The true efficient cause of Freud's uncanny affect is the 'certain circumstance' under which the repressed is prompted to return—whatever entity or event sparks the return, to which the affect attaches itself .... But let me posit that the repressed can return entirely on its own. What allows it to do so is that neither *un-* entirely succeeds in its operation. First, repression (the negating *un-*) is an imperfect mechanism. It seeks to effect an absence or lack but can never entirely divest us of something that belongs to us. It is always possible for this privation to be undone or reversed. That is, it is always possible for the reversing-releasing *un-* to spring into operation, undoing the repression. But, second, the reversing-releasing *un-* does not operate perfectly either. What is repressed is not simply unveiled; the *unheimlich* secret is revealed or released *as a secret*. The *un-* does not bring the secret fully into the open, overcoming hiddenness or concealment. It only makes the concealment manifest as such. This is why, finally, this revelation is disruptive: it introduces something still unfamiliar into the familiar. So what drives or permits the arising of the uncanny affect is the imperfect operation of both *un-*'s.
>
> The familiar is never fully repressed and the repressed is never fully revealed.
>
> *(Withy 218–19)*

She adds a pertinent footnote (219 n. 22):

> There is of course more to be said about why this is so. Thus Anneleen Masschelein explains it slightly differently: "The prefix 'un-' is not merely a linguistic negation, it is the 'token of repression'. This entails that the uncanny is marked by the unconscious that does not know negation or contradiction; even when something is negated, it still remains present in the unconscious. According to this reasoning, the contradiction resulting from negation is not exclusive or binary: denying something at the same time conjures it up." Anneleen Masschelein, *The Unconcept: The Freudian Uncanny in Late-Twentieth-Century Theory* (State University of New York Press, 2011), 8; see also 36.

In addition to the usual modalities in which unconscious material is made manifest, however obliquely—dreams, parapraxes, artistic creation, successful psychoanalytic therapy, and so on—Withy adds another, bound up with the very character of the mechanisms of repression and de-repression. But first it is worth recalling that parapraxes include not just slips of the tongue but other sorts of "error." In the

APA Dictionary of Psychology, a parapraxis is "an error that is believed to express unconscious wishes, attitudes, or impulses. Examples of such errors include slips of the pen, slips of the tongue and other forms of verbal leakage, forgetting significant events, mislaying objects with unpleasant associations, unintentional puns, and motivated accidents" (https://dictionary.apa.org/parapraxis). Freud himself ("The 'Uncanny'" 11) recalls an uncanny moment when his hasty effort to leave a street of prostitution in an Italian town into which he has wandered issues in two further "involuntary" returns to "the same street"—an instance of what we might term "ambulatory parapraxis." To return to Withy: the repressed, in her account, returns not as a recovered original—in the pristine condition of its pre-repressed status—but as something marked by its having been hidden before returning. In doing so, it "retains its unfamiliar character" but also "destabilizes the realm of the familiar" (Withy 216). The difference is something like that between an unsent letter in an envelope and that envelope brought back by a postal worker and marked "Return to Sender." It is once again here, but it is marked as having gone away before returning.

The metaphoric counterpart to this description of the psychoanalytic uncanny is of course different. Unlike Withy's repressed material, the metaphoric vehicle doesn't "return" from its cultural-linguistic cache, nor is it marked by its having been hidden (repressed). Rather, it emerges from a boundless and as yet unrealized cultural reservoir marked with the taboo of virtuality because it has been part of a forbidden (latent, unrealized, unauthorized) collection of verbal-conceptual signs. It is not merely a new name or label or even a newly-created entity, but a sign that has been culturally unavailable—thus metaphorically "forbidden"—by virtue of its latent or virtual status. Instead of being repressed—thrust into an individual unconscious at some point in the past—it exists at a threshold of *future* emergence, having undergone what might be termed "prevenient banishment." The difference is between the uncanny of the individual return of the repressed and the uncanny of the cultural imminence of the future: between the shock of the present exhumation of the bygone and the shock of the advent of the not-yet. More particularly, just as there is a necessary link between the uncanny and the return of the repressed—in Freud's formulation, "everything that is uncanny" emerges from the [return of] "repressed infantile complexes" or from "primitive beliefs [we believe] we have surmounted" (Freud, "The 'Uncanny'" 15, 17)—so there is a similar link between the emergence of the uncanny and the dynamics of the relation between tenor and vehicle in metaphor. Indeed, metaphor already implies the uncanny—the irrational, or at least the non-logical—in its founding, non-negotiable, and "scandalous" claim that one thing is another thing. The dimension of the uncanny is something that, so to speak, is not imposed on metaphoric structure but unfolds from within it.

Social Ritual and the Metaphoric Uncanny

Another perspective on the socio-cultural rather than individual dimension of metaphor is provided by the sphere of ritual and its attendant modes of uncanniness. In her brilliant study, *Purity and Danger: An Analysis of Concepts of Pollution and Taboo*, Mary Douglas notes that pollution rituals usually seek to isolate and expel forces that threaten cultural rules, categories, and order—as Girard also points out in his discussion of ritual sacrifice and scapegoating, *Violence and the Sacred.* But Douglas goes on to explain that certain rituals have a precisely contrary aim: the purposeful incorporation of threatening and potentially chaotic forces that, in addition to their destructiveness, nonetheless also hold the possibility of cultural transformation and growth. Consequently, at times these forces must not be expelled but ritually internalized if their power is to be harnessed to invigorate an overly rigid system of cultural norms and categories. The Lele people of the Congo, for example, normally regard the pangolin or scaly anteater with horror because it symbolizes the pollution associated with cross-categorial contamination: it is scaly like a fish, yet climbs trees; it looks like a lizard, yet it suckles its young like a mammal; and so on. It is a horror, an "other," a confounder of socio-cultural categories and therefore an instance of the uncanny. (In the third chapter of *Purity and Danger*, "The Abominations of Leviticus," Douglas explains how Old Testament dietary restrictions and taboos are also based on regarding categorial mingling as a mode of impurity.)

But at other times, this "hybrid monster" is ritually and "reverently eaten by initiates and taken to be the most powerful source of fertility," an introjected power capable of revivifying the schemata by which this society customarily lives (Douglas 168). Such rituals, with their attendant dangers, allow people to become aware of—rather than passively live within—those heretofore invisible constraints. Douglas generalizes powerfully from this example:

> Granted that disorder spoils pattern, it also provides the material of pattern. Order implies restriction; from all possible materials, a limited selection has been made and from all possible relations a limited set has been used. So disorder by implication is unlimited, no pattern has been realised in it, but its potential for patterning is indefinite. This is why, though we seek to create order, we do not simply condemn disorder. We recognise that it is destructive to existing patterns; also that it has potentiality. It symbolises both danger and power. Ritual recognises the potency of disorder. In dreams, faints and frenzies, ritual expects to find powers and truths which cannot be reached by conscious effort.
>
> *(Douglas 94)*

Disorder is a threat but also a possibility; its danger and power are also agents of change, permitting us to diminish the rigidity of the cultural system it otherwise threatens so directly and starkly. It is what Jacques Derrida calls a pharmakon: both sickness and cure, poison and antidote. (See Derrida, "Plato's Pharmacy" 63–171.) Like one form of apotropaic phenomena or rituals, it "wards off" evil but does so by reproducing or embodying that evil. In medical terms, it is a homeopathic rather than an allopathic agent. It "cures and infects" and is, in Jonathan Culler's words, "the element in which opposites are opposed, the movement and play by which each relates back to the other, reverses itself and passes into the other" (Culler, *On Deconstruction* 142–3).

Which is to say that disorder is uncanny—according to Jentsch's definition, Withy's, and even Freud's, so long as we remember that the Lele ritual is socio-cultural rather than individual, that the pangolin's taboo status serves as the collective counterpart to individual repression, and that the return of the repressed is performed metaphorically by the initiates' reverent ingestion of this "hybrid monster." "The Lele pangolin cult," Douglas continues,

> is only one example …. of cults which invite their initiates to turn round and confront the categories on which their whole surrounding culture has been built up and to recognise them for the fictive, man-made, arbitrary creations that they are … . By the mystery of that rite they recognise something of the fortuitous and conventional nature of the categories in whose mould they have their experience.

Put more generally, this rite "suggests a meditation on the inadequacy of the categories of human thought" (Douglas 170–1, 174)

It is something of a leap, but the structure and dynamics of metaphor can be thought of as a kind of socio-linguistic counterpart to the Lele pangolin ritual, a counterpart in which conventional linguistic-conceptual reality (roughly, "usage"), the sphere of the metaphoric tenor, corresponds to the orderly culture of the Lele people; the maker or receiver (roughly, "writer or reader") of the metaphor corresponds to the initiates of the pangolin cult who participate in the ritual; and the vehicle—once it is permitted to emerge into actuality from the virtual vastness of the as-yet-unrealized—corresponds to the pangolin: uncanny, pharmakon-like, chaotic, disruptive and destructive, but also potentially liberating and transformative of conventional socio-cultural reality and its sustaining but rigid and unyielding regularities and usages. The vehicles of a metaphor disorder our vocabulary, our signs—both the signifiers that designate concepts and the concepts thus designated. They may remain marginal and peripheral, even to the point of fading or disappearing after they have escaped latency and become manifest and actual; coexist in uneasy tension with established tenors; or displace those tenors, surrendering their figurative status to create what are known as "dead metaphors," about which Nietzsche writes evocatively: "truths are illusions about which one has forgotten that this is what they are; metaphors which are worn out and without sensuous power; coins which have lost their pictures and now matter only as metal, no longer as coins" (*The Portable Nietzsche* 46–7).

But the other side of such disorder may also be a net gain for vocabulary and culture, transforming and revivifying both as the uncanny becomes assimilated—metaphorically, introjected—into the usage-governed word hoard of the society. Granted (to adapt Douglas' formulation) that the vehicle is disruptive, a bringer of chaos, a scourge of usage and of the thoughtless communicative ease that usage can enable. It is also a liberator, a source of linguistic and conceptual fertility, an enlarger of reality, and an agent that brings to consciousness the miraculousness and the fragility of the arbitrariness that links signifiers with signifieds to create linguistic and conceptual intelligibility. For that miraculous intelligibility is also a mechanism of confinement—not least because its status as circumference or trap or cage is not seeable or questionable from within the system. It is, to borrow a phrase from Fredric Jameson, a prison-house of language. As prisoners, "We cannot imagine life outside, cannot even, in our theoretical discussions, think our way out," as Jonathan Culler remarks (Culler, "Language and Knowledge" 3). Inhabiting a dwelling whose form and appearance we cannot describe or even discern is surely another instance of the uncanny.

10

METAPHOR AND AFFECT

The Uncanny, Paradox, Wonder, Religion

In the seventeenth century, Sir Thomas Browne defends the emotive dimension of religious belief in *Religio Medici*: "I am, I confess, naturally inclined to that which misguided zeal terms superstition." Three centuries later, Rudolf Otto's *The Idea of the Holy* insists on "*the non-rational factor in the idea of the divine*." Otto's holy is radically unfamiliar, "wholly other," uncanny. Not that paradox, the uncanny, or metaphor are religious phenomena—only that the affective, the ineffable, and the suprarational overlap as in a Venn diagram.

Such notions of paradox, wonder, and religion follow from the initial assumption that metaphors are assertions of identity both true and false, constituting an "affront" to purity. But a functional, *productive* impurity is capable of achieving expressive and rhetorical ends unavailable to simpler or "purer" discourse.

In addition to these structural analogies and linkages, and the cognitive experiences they imply, there is a significant affective dimension to the reading or hearing or processing of metaphor—a dimension that is also inescapably uncanny. The mysteriousness of metaphor, its singularity and oddness, its simultaneous rightness and wrongness, truth and falsity, its striking aptness and surd-like unassimilability, its force of definitional trauma or definitional pleasure, even *jouissance*—these are experiences registered in various ways by many of the significant writers on metaphor on whom this inquiry has depended: Walker Percy, Kenneth Burke, Paul Ricoeur, Denis Donoghue, William Empson, Wallace Stevens, Hans Blumenberg, Nelson Goodman, and others. Such experiences require an account of metaphor that includes the language, concepts, and affect of the uncanny. In one of Jacques Rancière's formulations, metaphor is a paradoxical figure. It is, first, "a power of both order and disorder." Somewhat more specifically, it "brings together distant objects and makes their coming-together speak" but "also undoes the laws

DOI: 10.4324/9781003560050-10

of representation" (Rancière 159). These two dimensions of metaphor—the simultaneous management of order and disorder, and of articulate representation and the undoing of representation—are at once paradoxical and uncanny, and readerly experience of them is inevitably both cognitive and affective.

The paradoxical and the uncanny, moreover, have a long intertwinement with the experience of wonder. In the first place, the uncanny is clearly a special case or sub-category of the paradoxical and the self-contradictory. In the second, paradox is historically associated not just with self-contradiction but with self-contradiction *as a trope for the ineffable*, a way of gesturing toward that which cannot be wholly contained or expressed by ordinary, non-paradoxical language. Thus the object of certain rituals, insists Victor Turner, is "to use paradox and contradiction to express truths which are inexpressible in any other terms" (as paraphrased by Douglas, 176–7, without page reference, from Turner). That last phrase suggests truths that do not just evade or escape rational discourse but *exceed* it—that transcend common categories of reason and graspability. To take a parallel from the sphere of literary criticism, the eleventh chapter of Cleanth Brooks's *The Well Wrought Urn* is titled "The Heresy of Paraphrase"—where "paraphrase" signifies a reductive and even logocentric rhetoric—while the first chapter is approvingly titled "The Language of Paradox." This interest in paradox and the untranslatable, in turn, explains one frequent emotional response to metaphor: a fascination with the conceptual "beyond" (statements at once true and false, for example), and an insistence on non-paraphrasability: of much literary language in general ("A poem should not mean/But be," as Archibald MacLeish famously declared), of literary tropes as such, and especially of metaphor itself (MacLeish 106–7). Thus Max Black, in his rigorous and intellectually skeptical essay, "Metaphor," nonetheless speaks respectfully of "the secret and the mystery of metaphor" (Black, "Metaphor" 286).

The association of paradox and wonder has a long history. "Because of a tradition linking wonder to knowledge that goes back at least as far as Aristotle's *Metaphysics*," writes Peter G. Platt, "the paradoxical is also linked to wonder and the marvelous" (Platt, "'The Meruailouse [sic] Site'" n. pag. par. 12). Thus in the Renaissance, Platt observes, "we find George Puttenham speaking of '*Paradoxon*, or the Wondrer [wonderer],' and elaborating with an example: 'Many times our Poet is caried by some occasion to report of a thing that is maruelous, and then he will seeme not to speake it simply but with some signe of admiration [cf. Latin *admirari*: 'to wonder at']'" (Puttenham 189). "John Florio's Italian-English dictionary of 1598, A Worlde of Wordes," Platt continues, defines paradox as "'a maruellous, wonderfull and strange thinge to heare'" (Platt par. 12). And Francesco Patrizi, a sixteenth-century anti-Aristotelian humanist, noted that "'the marvelous is always paradox'" (Platt par. 13). Many readers' responses to the uncanny, and to metaphor, derive in part from this special valuation of paradox and contradiction, from the association of paradox with that which is puzzling, confusing, or confounding and also with values beyond system, rationality, and traditional logic (and rhetoric).

The pervasiveness of the historical valorization of paradox is very recently attested to by Elizabeth S. Anker in *On Paradox: The Claims of Theory*, in which Anker explores but also critiques the association of paradox with value, lamenting the seductions she believes it has exerted on humanistic and critical thought. Of course, paradox itself has frequently been seen as an agent of demystification and cultural critique. Platt notes that Rosalie Colie's book on Renaissance paradox, *Paradoxia Epidemica: The Renaissance Tradition of Paradox*,

> has highlighted paradox's role in undoing certainty and conventional wisdom. The figure inevitably involves an "exploitation of the fact of relative, or competing, value systems. The paradox is always somehow involved in dialectic: challenging some orthodoxy, the paradox is an oblique criticism of absolute judgment or absolute convention."
>
> *(Platt par. 12)*

The mention of competing value systems recalls Douglas' remark about cultural categories as "fictive, man-made, arbitrary creations," as well as Withy's linking of the uncanny with "an irresolvable uncertainty about the applicability of the very categories that we use." The uncanny object must be "radically anomalous, in the sense that it calls the jointing of our 'ideational sphere' into question" (Withy 18).

Affect and Religious Paradox

Such power of critique, seeming to lay bare the creation or production of what had been taken as simply and unquestionably given—to translate, paradoxically, the natural into the cultural—edges toward another sphere of discourse in which a new and startling world view founded on paradox offers to contend with the conventional and more readily comprehensible values of the contemporary society: the discourse of religion. As Douglas remarks, "any ritual which expresses the happy union of opposites is also an apt vehicle for essentially religious themes" (Douglas 170). Particularly apt for religions like Christianity that are fundamentally grounded on "heterodox" ideas such as that the last shall be first, that to find one's life one must first lose it, that it is possible to be wholly human and wholly divine at the same moment, and that the Fall of humankind was simultaneously an occasion for death and for eternal life—a *felix culpa* or lucky guilt, or fortunate fall, or auspicious crime. As the narrator of T. S. Eliot's "The Journey of the Magi" muses, puzzled and "no longer at ease" in the presence of mystery:

> were we led all that way for
> Birth or Death? There was a Birth, certainly,
> We had evidence and no doubt. I had seen birth and death,

But had thought they were different; this Birth was
Hard and bitter agony for us, like Death, our death.

In the mid-seventeenth century, noted above, Sir Thomas Browne mounts a shrewd, characteristically witty, and highly rational defense of the more-than-rational dimension of religious belief in his *Religio Medici*. He announces: "I am, I confess, naturally inclined to that which misguided zeal terms superstition" (Browne 1571). It is notable that he terms his "superstition" a natural rather than a wayward or perverse inclination, and that he reserves language critical of the irrational and "enthusiastic" (in the older sense of "uncritically approving") for those *skeptical* of his inclination: unlike Browne himself, they are creatures of "misguided zeal." He elaborates this attitude toward faith and reason in a famous passage:

> Methinks there be not impossibilities enough in religion for an active faith … I love to lose myself in a mystery, to pursue my Reason to an *O altitudo!* … I can answer all the objections of Satan and my rebellious reason with that odd resolution I learned of Tertullian, *Certum est quia impossibile est* [It is certain *because* it is impossible].
>
> *(Browne 1574. Most modern scholarship rejects the attribution to Tertullian. See Harrison.)*

This delicate management of the rational and the irrational—in effect, a rational defense of the irrational—is carried on, theorized, and argued at length in the early twentieth century by Rudolf Otto in *The Idea of the Holy: An Inquiry into the Non-Rational Factor in the Idea of the Divine and Its Relation to the Rational.* Otto's insistence on the affective dimension of faith appears in the very first line of his epigraph from Goethe: "Das Schaudern ist der Menschheit bestes Teil." *The shudder is the best part of humanity.* Like Browne, Otto requires no absolute choice between rational knowledge and the irrational; as noted, his project is to constitute a reasonable defense of the latter. The experience he describes in his study is a form of "genuine 'knowing,'" though in contrast to ordinary or rational knowing it may be termed "non-rational" (Otto, translator's preface x–xi). Rather than a complete flight from rationality, the holy is rather "a fabric in which we have the non-rational numinous experience as the woof and the rational and ethical as the warp" (Otto, translator's preface xiii). Nonetheless, the holy is radically foreign, unfamiliar, distressing, at times unintelligible—in short, uncanny. In one of the book's foundational and best-known phrases, Otto identifies the mysterious as "the wholly other" [*Das ganz Andere*]. It is beyond "the usual, the intelligible, and the familiar … outside the limits of the 'canny,'" and it fills the mind "with blank wonder and astonishment" (the aesthetic category of the sublime is clearly a close relative of Otto's holy). Encountering the wholly other, "we recoil in a wonder that strikes us chill and numb" (Otto 26, 28).

This is obviously not to claim that paradox, or the uncanny, or metaphor itself is a religious phenomenon—nor even to intimate that they cast what Milton, in *Il Penseroso*, calls "a dim religious light." Only that the power so often associated with these phenomena has a counterpart in the vocabulary of religious paradox and religious mystery, and that this fact suggests that the affective charge, the sense of wonder, the incomprehensibility, the ineffable and untranslatable, the supra-rational, and the transcendent overlap like the circles of a Venn diagram with paradox at its center:

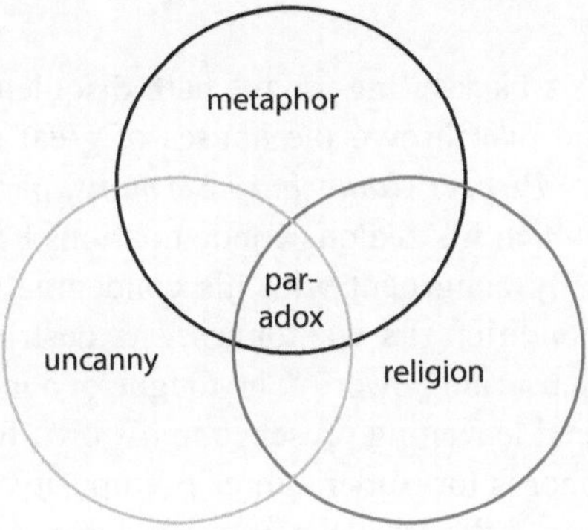

It is worth recalling that these claims about paradox, wonder, the ineffable, and so on, and about religious discourse and modes of the non-rational, all derive from our initial assumption that metaphors are not comparisons but assertions of identity—thus at once true and false. To quote Butler one last time, "Every thing is what it is, and not another thing," a remark reminding us that the paradoxical character of metaphoric operation provokes readerly resistance ranging from hesitation and puzzlement to categorial outrage. That outrage, often enough, derives from a sense of violation, trespass, and impurity in the face of metaphoric assertions or of comparable ontological challenges such as (once again) Woolf's "nothing was simply one thing."

Metaphor and Impurity

The link between outrage and the affront of impurity appears in Butler's own rhetoric, where he himself has recourse—perhaps surprisingly, perhaps not—to metaphorical language in order to condemn the waywardness and alien toxicity of intemperate speech. In "Sermon IV. Upon the Government of the Tongue," he laments that

> There is in some such a disposition to be talking, that an offence of the slightest kind, and such as would not raise any other resentment, yet raises, if I may so

> speak, *the resentment of the tongue, puts it into a flame, into the most ungovernable motions.* [Men] have not a due government over their tongue.
>
> *(par. 5)*

> And this *unrestrained volubility, and wantonness of speech* … begets resentment in him who is the subject of it; sows the seed of strife and dissension amongst others; and inflames little disgusts and offences, which, if let alone, would wear away of themselves.
>
> *(par. 7)*

Butler concludes with "'A back-biting tongue hath disquieted many; strong cities hath it pulled down, and overthrown the houses of great men. *The tongue of a man is his fall*'" (Butler, *Project Canterbury Sermons*, par. 21). Butler's implicit rejection of metaphor, which his zealous condemnations here override or at least complicate, is structurally congruent with his condemnation of an ungoverned tongue—its inflamed condition, its wantonness, its destruction of cities and of great men's houses, its lapsarian power: "The tongue of a man is his fall." Despite its inescapable and indeed leavening presence in his own frequently abstract and desiccated prose, metaphor is for Butler a force of impurity, implicitly linked with an ungoverned tongue. In different ways, metaphor and a wayward tongue taint the discourses of which they are part, discourses whose homogeneity is violated, for Butler, by the alien otherness of ungoverned speech and by the alogical and ontologically incoherent figure of metaphor. "Purity and Danger" indeed, to borrow Mary Douglas' title.

11
CONCLUSION

The Uses of Impurity

Impurity, however, can take many forms, some destructive and debilitating, others inconsequential, yet still others productive and salutary. A pathogen introduced into a living body may injure that body or destroy its life. But in another form, that pathogen can become an inoculatory agent, a vaccine, that works to preserve health and life. Recall the earlier discussion of the *pharmakon*, apotropaic defensive agents, and Douglas' exploration of the dual and self-contradictory nature of the pangolin: a taboo creature of profoundly destructive otherness but also—once ritually introjected—a source of fertility displaying what Mikkel Borch-Jacobsen terms "an intimate otherness" (Borch-Jacobsen 6). This notion of impurity is what I would like to offer as a final context for metaphor: a fertile impurity that makes possible a complexity of great power and interest by sacrificing purity, simplicity, homogeneity, immaculateness, pristine unity for conceptual, linguistic, and ontological depth, richness, and endless interpretability. (I will remark, in passing, that Jonathan Swift's writings conduct a sustained, satiric critique of an idealized conception of purity, as in "Cassinus and Peter: A Tragical Elegy" and numerous other texts.)

The aesthetic dimensions of purity and impurity, for example, are a principal subject of Plotinus' *Enneads* as lucidly explicated by W. K. Wimsatt (Wimsatt & Brooks 113–18. Wimsatt notes that "The Works of Plotinus are quoted … from the translation of Stephen MacKenna, 5 vols., London, 1917–30, by permission of Faber and Faber Limited and Pantheon Books Inc."). Plotinus distinguishes between two forms of beauty, which we can loosely label pure and impure, and which correspond to the two meanings Plotinus ascribes to the word "simple" (*haplous*). In Wimsatt's words,

DOI: 10.4324/9781003560050-11

> We have seen that the emphasis of the Plotinian system lies upon a kind of unity which we can conceive as the triumph of an ordering principle over multiplicity and diversity of parts. It is even difficult to conceive this triumph except as occurring through and in virtue of the diversity of the parts. The Plotinian term "simple" (*haplous*) … may describe either *absence* of *internal differentiation* (as with the simplicity or unity of a pebble) or precisely the opposite, a high degree of *internal differentiation*—in other words, organic unity (as with the unity of a living body).
>
> *(Wimsatt & Brooks 118)*

Plotinus elaborates elsewhere: "[T]here is the beauty, conferred by craftsmanship, of … a house with all its parts, and the beauty which some natural quality may give to a single stone" (Plotinus, *Ennead* 1.6.2). And at greater length in *Ennead* 5.8.1:

> Suppose two blocks of stone lying side by side: one is unpatterned, quite untouched by art; the other has been minutely wrought by the craftsman's hands into some statue of God or man, a Grace or a Muse, or if a human being, not a portrait but a creation in which the sculptor's art has concentrated all loveliness.
>
> Now it must be seen that the stone thus brought under the artist's hand to the beauty of form is beautiful not as stone—for so the crude stone would be as pleasant—but in virtue of the form or idea introduced by art. This form is not in the material; it is in the designer before it enters the stone.
>
> *(Wimsatt & Brooks 122)*

The first sort of beauty, which I am terming "pure," is that of a simple, undifferentiated, and internally homogeneous object. Purely, and merely, stone all the way through: a single whole object—no parts or divisions. The second or "impure" mode of beauty—that of a stone statue rather than a stone—is complex rather than simple, of multiple parts and thus internally differentiated, and its unity is thus a multiform and heterogeneous unity deriving from the numerous interrelations of part to part and part to whole. Interest, novelty, maturity of vision, complex rather than simple truths, tension, even self-contradiction—these may be had only by forgoing monolithic purity for multiform impurity.

An analogous distinction appears—in a moral and religious rather than an aesthetic context—in a central passage of Milton's defense of the liberty of unlicensed printing, *Areopagitica.* "I cannot praise a fugitive and cloister'd vertue," he begins, "unexercis'd & unbreath'd, that never sallies out and sees her adversary, but slinks out of the race, where that immortall garland is to be run for, not without dust and heat." He concludes this portion of his argument with a distinction almost exactly parallel to that between Plotinus' pure and impure unity. "That vertue therefore which is but a youngling in the contemplation of evill, and knows not the utmost that vice promises to her followers, and rejects it, is but a *blank vertue, not a pure*" (Milton, *Areopagitica* n. pag., my italics). In Milton's vocabulary, a "blank" virtue aligns with Plotinus' notion of simple and undifferentiated beauty, stone rather than statue, while a "pure" virtue corresponds to Plotinus' conception of complex and internally differentiated beauty (in Milton's argument that means a virtue willing to submit to trial by its opposite: "knowing good and evill, that is to say … knowing good by evill. As therefore the state of man now is; what wisdome can there be to choose, what continence to forbeare without the knowledge of evill?"). In both Plotinus and Milton, the tried and mature wisdom that transcends the "blank" simplicity of a "youngling" is unreachable without the impurity that only complexity makes possible.

Examples of this sort of paradoxical structure, of an impurity that transcends what Plotinus calls unpatterned and artless beauty and Milton "a blank virtue," are numerous in Western literary and philosophical discourse, early and late. Yeats's poem, "Crazy Jane Talks with The Bishop," for example, pits the Bishop's conventional and orthodox opposition between the spiritual and the corporeal, soul and body, against Jane's insistent refusal to separate these terms or spheres:

I met the Bishop on the road
And much said he and I.
"Those breasts are flat and fallen now
Those veins must soon be dry;
Live in a heavenly mansion,
Not in some foul sty."

"Fair and foul are near of kin,
And fair needs foul," I cried.
"My friends are gone, but that's a truth
Nor grave nor bed denied,
Learned in bodily lowliness
And in the heart's pride.

"A woman can be proud and stiff
When on love intent;
But Love has pitched his mansion in
The place of excrement;
For nothing can be sole or whole
That has not been rent."

For Jane, truths are learned not in abstract elevation or "a heavenly mansion," and not in the humility of age, but in "bodily lowliness" and "the heart's pride." Love (capital "L"), whether an idealization, an abstraction, or a personification, has "pitched his mansion in/The place of excrement"—that corporeal region scandalously shared by the genital and the excretory—as Christ lovingly "pitched" his divinity in the place of decay and death: the human body. Speaking of what he terms "*the incredible condescension of the Incarnation*," Gerard Manley Hopkins remarks that "our Lord submitted not only to the pains of life, the fasting, scourging, crucifixion etc. or the insults, as the mocking, blindfolding, spitting etc., but also to *the mean and trivial accidents of humanity*" (Hopkins, *Further Letters* 19–20). Compare the discussion of *felix culpa*, above (p. 85), as well as a quotation uncertainly attributed to St. Augustine of Hippo (AD 354–430), which offers a similar bodily paradox: "*Inter faeces et urinam nascimur*"—*we are born amidst feces and urine*. In a jarring passage, directly contrary to the Bishop's orthodox dichotomies, Jane cries that "Fair and foul are near of kin,/And fair needs foul" (monosyllables and alliteration reinforce the links between the traditionally distinct and antithetical "fair" and "foul"), and she claims even more dramatically in the final lines that "Nothing can be sole or whole/That has not been rent" (lines 7–8, 17–18). For something to possess authentic solitude and separateness, wholeness and completeness, it must be torn, invaded, and violated.

This is not simply a literary or an artistic phenomenon. In the biological world, to take just one instance, an organic version of one sort of purity is found in the status of an unfertilized egg: sole, whole, internally relatively undifferentiated—a seeming exemplar of uniformity and self-containedness. But once that solitary integrity—"blank," Milton might have termed it—is disrupted by an entering sperm cell that breaches its boundary, the egg begins to divide, progressively, until the many distinct cells produced by internal differentiation create a complex system of relationships to one another. This process results in a different—a Plotinian—kind of wholeness from that of the unfertilized egg: not a blank, living cell but a richly individuated animal or person, sole and whole in an entirely different—and more highly valued—way than the unviolated egg.

In this connection, Jane's epithet, "Crazy," may recall not simply the condition of being foolish, unconventional, or mentally unsound but also another kind of "crackedness": "Full of cracks or flaws; liable to break or fall to pieces; rickety; dilapidated," which in turn is sometimes used in the form "crazed" as applied to pottery: 'On the table was ... a beautiful crazed ceramic jug of blue and yellow flowers'" (*OED*, s.v. "crazed" 1.b). The jug is "crazed," but also "beautiful," or *and* also beautiful, a suitable vessel for cut flowers, in part because crazing became a prized artistic effect after it was initially regarded as merely a defect or flaw: a valued aesthetic condition that is made possible only by its first being a mode of injury or defect or fragmentation or impurity.

Finally, what is said of metaphor in this book appears in a more general context of truth-telling—not only poetic or literary—in the lyric by Emily Dickinson with which it began, "Tell all the truth but tell it slant." The poem is a potent argument for and an example of functional, productive impurity, capable of achieving expressive and rhetorical ends unavailable to directness or simplicity or purity of discourse. Only such a strategy can attain to the truths that directness cannot reach, can "By indirections find directions out," can illuminate or enlighten by paradoxically taming lightning's power to blind, can tell by "slant" what cannot be told straight, and can attain to truth by means of a "Circuit" that not only eschews directness but additionally—paradoxically, magically—identifies the "Success" of telling "all the truth" with the fact that "Success" also "lies." This account of functional, productive, potentially profound discursive impurity also describes the nature and power of that most compelling of figures of speech, metaphor.

APPENDIX

Below is a brief summary of the valuable account of four principal views of metaphor in M. H. Abrams and Geoffrey Galt Harpham, *A Glossary of Literary Terms* (s.v. "metaphor, theories of," pp. 213–16). The reader is encouraged to consult the entirety of Abrams' instructive entry.

In the opening paragraph of his concise account of theory of metaphor, M. H. Abrams notes that "there is no general agreement about the way we identify metaphors, how we are able to understand them, and what (if anything) they serve to tell us." He then offers "a brief summary of the most prominent among competing theories of metaphor":

First is "the similarity view." Introduced by Aristotle in the fourth century BC and still influential, the similarity view sees metaphor as a figurative rather than literal use of language; it works like a simile, offering an implicit comparison of two distinct things. This view treats metaphor as mainly a rhetorical enhancement of language, reducible without much loss of meaning to the literal statement it renders more vivid, or striking, or more satisfyingly "literary." It takes an overtly comparative simile—"their marriage is like a contact sport," say—and changes it to an *implicit* comparison in the form of a direct statement of identity: "Their marriage is a contact sport."

The second or "interactive" view of metaphor is associated with I. A. Richards who (in *The Philosophy of Rhetoric*, 1936) proposed the terms "tenor" and "vehicle" for the two parts of a metaphor (for example, "life" and "bowl of cherries"), and replaced the "similarity view" with a theory of *interaction* between the two terms. That often complex interaction is not reducible to the simile-like comparison of the first view. In addition, this view regards metaphor as not merely an enhancement or prettification of ordinary language but as a discursive and conceptual mode that, in Abrams' words, "permeates all language and affects the ways we perceive and conceive the world."

In his important essay "Metaphor" (1954–55), philosopher Max Black elaborated and extended Richards' approach, seeing tenor and vehicle as each possessing "a system of associated commonplaces"—features and relations that are regularly seen as linked with each element. In "The senate is a barnyard," for instance, "senate" traditionally implies human governance, elevated social rank, public service and aims, reasoned debate and orderly procedures, and more. A "barnyard," on the other hand, implies various forms and species of animal, an emphasis on bodily survival and satisfaction, limited social vision or organization, conflict resolution not by debate but by physical intimidation or self-inhibited aggression (a posture of subordination), no humanly speechlike communication, and an orderly schedule based on physical needs (food, sleep, etc.) and the strictures imposed by human caretakers. The interpreter's selection from each of these clusters of association will determine what the metaphor is suggesting about its two principal entities and their relations. (Compare Todorov's conception of metaphor as double synecdoche, p. 7 above.) Black also reminds us that a metaphor is not simply unidirectional. "If to call a man a wolf is to put him in a special light, we must not forget that the metaphor makes the wolf seem more human than he otherwise would" (Black, "Metaphor" 291). And he observes that while we often assume that metaphors call attention to a pre-existing similarity between two entities, "it would be more illuminating in some of these cases to say that the metaphor *creates* the similarity" (284–5, my italics).

In a sharp turn, philosopher Donald Davidson ("What Metaphors Mean," 1978, 32) contends that there is *no* metaphorical meaning separate from literal meaning. Abrams terms this—his third category—"the pragmatic view," indicating a focus on what the metaphor *does* rather than what it *means* (the "semantic" view). Metaphors, Davidson argues, "mean what the words, in their most literal interpretation, mean, and nothing more." The metaphoric import of a phrase or sentence *may lead the reader to discover or entertain* something about the relations between the two terms. If "The senate is a barnyard," for example, is a literal and not a figurative or metaphorical assertion, what does it encourage or permit us to see as the connections between the two terms? The creator of the metaphor makes a literal claim about the identity of two different things: "Time is money," for instance. The interpreter infers or develops or constructs from this literal claim a metaphoric meaning that the (literal) metaphor enables but does not itself produce or express.

Abrams' fourth and final category, "the cognitive (or conceptual) view," sees ordinary discourse as itself powerfully and inescapably metaphorical in that it offers an extensive array of common conceptual categories or assertions or images: life as a journey; a developing person or intellectual movement as a growing plant; mental ignorance as physical blindness; a heated difference of opinion as a battle, or as war; height as a form of goodness, and depth as the corresponding sphere of badness ("The superb heights to which she has risen" versus "The sordid depths to which he has sunk"). Proponents of the cognitive or conceptual theory of metaphor seek to chart the powerful conceptual structures and their attendant values that shape human discourse and human thought, even entire societies, although we may rarely be aware of them. For several critiques of this school's attention to ideas and concepts but not to the language that conveys, expresses, and shapes those concepts, see above, pp. 3–4.

Indeed, the present study does not fit tidily into any one of the categories that Abrams describes though it does align itself principally with the second or "interaction" view of metaphor and to some extent with the third or "pragmatic" view. It is also resolutely committed to the *linguistic* dimension of metaphor and understands the conceptual or cognitive as inescapably expressed and fundamentally shaped by its linguistic form.

BIBLIOGRAPHY

Abrams, M. H., and Geoffrey Galt Harpham. *A Glossary of Literary Terms*, 11th edition. Cengage Learning, 2015.

Ambrose, Saint. *Expositio euangelii secundum Lucam 7.134; Commentary of Saint Ambrose on the Gospel according to Saint Luke*. Translated by Íde M. Ní Riain. Halcyon, 2001.

Anker, Elizabeth S. *On Paradox: The Claims of Theory*. Duke University Press, 2022.

Aristotle on Rhetoric: A Theory of Civic Discourse. Translated by George A. Kennedy, 2nd edition. Oxford University Press, 2007.

Auden, W. H. *Collected Poems*. Edited by Edward Mendelson. Random House, 1976.

Auerbach, Erich. "Figura." Erich Auerbach. *Scenes from the Drama of European Literature*. University of Minnesota Press, 1984, pp. 9–76.

Augustine, of Hippo, Saint, 354–430. *Nicene and Post-Nicene Fathers: Series I* (1885). Alexander Roberts and James Donaldson (original translators and editors); Arthur Cleveland Coxe (editor of American edition, unauthorized; and author of annotations, notes, and introductions); Philip Schaff (also credited as editor). https://en.wikisource.org/wiki/Nicene_and_Post-Nicene_Fathers:_Series_I/Volume_VII/Two_Books_of_Soliloquies/Book_II.

Barany, Michael. "Mathematical Ideality and the Practice of Translation." Unpublished paper, used by kind permission of the author, p. 16.

Barthes, Roland. *S/Z*. Translated by Richard Miller. Hill and Wang, 1974.

Beardsley, Monroe C. *Aesthetics*. Harcourt, Brace and World, 1958.

Belin, H. E. "The Civil War as Seen Through Southern Glasses." *American Journal of Sociology*, Vol. 9, No. 2, September 1903, pp. 259–67.

Berggren, Douglas. "The Use and Abuse of Metaphor, I." *The Review of Metaphysics*, Vol. 16, No. 2, December 1962, pp. 237–58.

Berggren, Douglas. "The Use and Abuse of Metaphor, II." *The Review of Metaphysics*, Vol. 16, No. 3, March 1963, pp. 450–72.

Black, Max. "Metaphor." *Proceedings of the Aristotelian Society, New Series*, Vol. 55, Issue 1, 1954–55, pp. 273–94.

Black, Max. *Models and Metaphors: Studies in Language and Philosophy.* Cornell University Press, 1962.

Blackmur, R. P. Review of Norman Macleod, *Horizons of Death. Poetry*, vol. 46, 1935, p. 108.

Blackwell, Mark, editor. *The Secret Life of Things: Animals, Objects, and It-Narratives in Eighteenth-Century England.* Bucknell University Press, 2007.

Blake, William. "*A Vision of the Last Judgment.*" *The Complete Poetry & Prose of William Blake*, newly revised edition, edited by David V. Erdman, commentary by Harold Bloom. Anchor Books, Doubleday, 1988, pp. 565–6.

Blumenberg, Hans. "Prospect for a Theory of Nonconceptuality." Hans Blumenberg, *Shipwreck with Spectator: Paradigm of a Metaphor for Existence.* Translated by Stephen Rendall. MIT Press, 1997, pp. 81–102.

Blumenberg, Hans. *Paradigms for a Metaphorology.* Translated from the German with an afterword by Robert Savage. Cornell University Press and Cornell University Library, 2010.

Bogel, Fredric. *The Difference Satire Makes: Rhetoric and Reading from Jonson to Byron.* Cornell University Press, 2001.

Bogel, Fredric. *New Formalist Criticism: Theory and Practice.* Palgrave Macmillan, 2013.

Borch-Jacobsen, Mikkel. *The Freudian Subject.* Translated by Catherine Porter. Stanford University Press, 1988.

Boswell James. *Life of Johnson.* Edited by R. W. Chapman. Oxford University Press, 1998.

Bresnick, Adam. "Prosopoetic Compulsion: Reading the Uncanny in Freud and Hoffmann." *Germanic Review*, Spring 1996, Vol. 71, No. 2, pp. 114–32.

Breton, André. *Les Vases Communicants.* Librairie Gallimard, 1955.

Breton, André. *Manifestoes of Surrealism.* Translated by Richard Seaver and Helen R. Lane. University of Michigan Press, 1969.

Brooke-Rose, Christine. *A Grammar of Metaphor.* Secker & Warburg, 1958.

Brooks, Cleanth. *The Well Wrought Urn: Studies in the Structure of Poetry.* Harcourt, 1947.

Browne, Sir Thomas. *Religio Medici. The Norton Anthology of English Literature*, 7th edition, vol. 1. Edited by M. H. Abrams, *et al.* W. W. Norton & Company, 2000, p. 1571.

Burke, Edmund. *Speech on a Motion Made in the House of Commons MAY 11, 1793 ... Upon the Occasion of A Petition of the Unitarian Society. The Works of the Right Honorable Edmund Burke in Twelve Volumes, Volume the Seventh.* John C. Nimmo, MDCCCLXXXVII.

Burke, Edmund. *Reflections on the Revolution in France.* Edited by L. G. Mitchell. Oxford University Press, 2009.

Burke, Kenneth. Appendix D, "Four Master Tropes." *A Grammar of Motives and A Rhetoric of Motives.* Meridian Books, 1962.

Burke, Kenneth. *Permanence and Change: An Anatomy of Purpose*, 3rd edition. University of California Press, 1984.

Butler, Bishop Joseph. *Project Canterbury Sermons. Fifteen Sermons Preached at the Rolls Chapel By Joseph Butler.* Cambridge: Hilliard and Brown; Boston: Hilliard, Gray, Little, and Wilkins, 1827. Transcribed by LeRoy Dagg, 2002. Reproduced with permission of the Bishop Payne Library, Virginia Theological Seminary, 2005, n. pag. Par. 39. http://anglicanhistory.org/butler/rolls/preface.html.

Carman, Taylor. Review of Katherine Withy, *Heidegger on Being Uncanny. European Journal of Philosophy*, Vol. 25, Issue 3, September 2017, pp. 899–903.

Caruth, Cathy. *Unclaimed Experience: Trauma, Narrative, and History.* Johns Hopkins University Press, 1996.

Cassirer, Ernst. *Language and Myth.* Translated by Susanne K. Langer. Harper & Brothers, 1946.

Coleridge, Samuel Taylor, "Idea of the Christian Church." *On the constitution of the Church and State according to the idea of each*, 3rd edition. William Pickering, 1839, pp. 126–7.

Colie, Rosalie L. *Paradoxia Epidemica: The Renaissance Tradition of Paradox.* Princeton University Press, 1966.

Culler, Jonathan. "Commentary." *New Literary History*, Vol. 6, No. 1, Autumn 1974, pp. 219–29.

Culler, Jonathan. *On Deconstruction: Theory and Criticism after Structuralism.* Cornell University Press, 1983.

Culler, Jonathan. *Ferdinand de Saussure*, revised edition. Cornell University Press, 1986.

Culler, Jonathan. "Language and Knowledge: Joint Review of Fredric Jameson's *The Prison-House of Language: A Critical Account of Structuralism and Russian Formalism* and Michel Foucault's *The Archeology of Knowledge.*" *Michel Foucault: Critical Assessments, Vol. II.* Edited by Barry Smart. Routledge, 1994, pp. 3–7.

Culler, Jonathan. *Literary Theory: A Very Short Introduction.* Oxford University Press, 1997.

Cureton, Richard D. "Metaphor without Analogy: Samuel R. Levin's *The Semantics of Metaphor.*" *Poetics Today*, Vol. 4, No. 2, 1983, pp. 323–41.

"Darmok." *Star Trek: The Next Generation.* Season 5, Episode 2. Original air date: 30 September 1991. See also *Wikipedia*, s.v. "Darmok." https://en.wikipedia.org/wiki/Darmok.

Davidson, Donald. "What Metaphors Mean." *Critical Inquiry.* Vol. 5, No. 1, Special Issue on Metaphor, Autumn 1978, pp. 31–47.

de Man, Paul. "The Crisis of Contemporary Criticism." *Arion: A Journal of Humanities and the Classics*, Vol. 6, No. 1, 1967, pp. 38–57.

de Man, Paul. "The Epistemology of Metaphor." *Critical Inquiry*, Vol. 5, No. 1, Special Issue on Metaphor, Autumn 1978, pp. 13–30.

Derrida, Jacques, and C. T. Moore. "White Mythology: Metaphor in the Text of Philosophy." *New Literary History*, Vol. 6, No. 1, *On Metaphor*, Autumn 1974, pp. 5–74.

Derrida, Jacques, and C. T. Moore. "Plato's Pharmacy." *Dissemination.* Translated by Barbara Johnson. University of Chicago Press, 1981, pp. 63–171.

Dickinson, Emily. *The Poems of Emily Dickinson: Reading Edition.* Edited by R. W. Franklin. The Belknap Press of Harvard University Press, 1999.

Donoghue, Denis. *Metaphor.* Harvard University Press, 2014.

Douglas, Mary. *Purity and Danger: An Analysis of Concepts of Pollution and Taboo.* Routledge, 1966.

Durham, Deborah, and James W. Fernandez. "Tropical Dominions: The Figurative Struggle over Domains of Belonging and Apartness in Africa." *Beyond Metaphor: The Theory of Tropes in Anthropology.* Edited by James W. Fernandez. Stanford University Press, 1991, pp. 190–210.

Eliot, T. S. "Tradition and the Individual Talent." *Selected Prose of T. S. Eliot.* Edited by Frank Kermode. Harvest Books, 1975, pp. 37–45.

Eliot, T. S. "The Journey of the Magi." *Collected Poems 1909–1962*. Faber & Faber, 2002, pp. 99–100.

Empson, William. *The Structure of Complex Words*. University of Michigan Press, 1967.

Engh, Line Cecilie. Review of "Kretschmer, Marek Thue, ed. *La typologie biblique comme forme de pensée dans l'historiographie médiévale*." *Journal of Medieval Latin*, Vol. 25, 2015, pp. 1–6.

Everett, Percival. *James: A Novel*. Doubleday, 2024.

Ferber, Michael. *Poetry and Language: The Linguistics of Verse*. Cambridge University Press, 2019.

Freud, Sigmund. "The 'Uncanny.'" First published in *Imago*, Bd. V., 1919; reprinted in *Sammlung, Fünfte Folge*. Translated by Alix Strachey.

Freud, Sigmund. "The 'Uncanny.'" https://web.mit.edu/allanmc/www/freud1/pdf.

Freud, Sigmund. "The 'Uncanny'" (1919). *Standard Edition of the Complete Psychological Works*, 24 vols. Edited and Translated by James Strachey, vol. 17. The Hogarth Press, 1953, pp. 217–53.

Freud, Sigmund. "Beyond the Pleasure Principle." *Standard Edition of the Complete Psychological Works*, 24 vols. Edited and Translated by James Strachey, vol. 18. The Hogarth Press, 1955, pp. 3–64.

Fried, Debra. "Repetition, Refrain, and Epitaph." *ELH*, Vol. 53, No. 3, Autumn 1986, pp. 615–32.

Frost, Robert. *Poems, Prose, & Plays*. Edited by Richard Poirier and Mark Richardson. Library of America, 1995.

Frye, Northrop. *Anatomy of Criticism: Four Essays*. Princeton University Press, 1957.

Gallie, W. B. "Essentially Contested Concepts." *Proceedings of the Aristotelian Society*, Vol. 56, 1956, pp. 167–98.

Girard, René. *Violence and the Sacred*. Translated by Patrick Flaherty. Johns Hopkins University Press, 1977.

Goodman, Nelson. *Languages of Art: An Approach to a Theory of Symbols*. Bobbs-Merrill, 1968.

Goodman, Nelson. "Metaphor as Moonlighting." *Critical Inquiry*, Vol. 6, No. 1, Autumn 1979, pp. 125–30.

Grice, Paul. *Studies in The Way of Words*. Harvard University Press, 1989.

Griffith, Susan Blackburn. "Unwrapping the Word: Metaphor in the Augustinian Imagination." *Studia Patristica* 70, vol. 18: *St Augustine and His Opponents*. Edited by Markus Vinzent. Peeters, 2013, pp. 213–20.

Harrison, Peter. "'I Believe Because It Is Absurd': The Enlightenment Invention of Tertullian's Credo." *Church History*, Vol. 86, No. 2, 2017, pp. 339–64.

Hertz, Neil. *The End of the Line: Essays on Psychoanalysis and the Sublime*. Columbia University Press, 1985.

Hester, Marcus B. *The Meaning of Poetic Metaphor: An Analysis in the Light of Wittgenstein's Claim That Meaning Is Use*. Mouton & Co., 1967.

Hills, David. "Metaphor." *The Stanford Encyclopedia of Philosophy* (Fall 2017 edition). Edited by Edward N. Zalta. https://plato.stanford.edu/archives/fall2017/entries/metaphor/.

Hoover Company, The. https://en.wikipedia.org/w/index.php?title=The_Hoover_Company&oldid=1073191310.

Hopkins, Gerard Manley. *Further Letters of Gerard Manley Hopkins*. Edited by Claude Colleer Abbott. Oxford University Press, 1956.

Hughes, Ted. *Collected Poems*. Edited by Paul Keegan. Farrar, Straus and Giroux, 2003.

Jakobson, Roman. "Closing Statement: Linguistics and Poetics." *Style in Language*. Edited by Thomas A. Sebeok. Technology Press of Massachusetts Institute of Technology and John Wiley & Sons, 1960, pp. 350–77.

Jarrell, Randall. *The Complete Poems.* Farrar, Straus and Giroux, 1981.

Jaynes, Julian. *The Origin of Consciousness in the Breakdown of the Bicameral Mind.* Houghton Mifflin, 1976.

Jaynes, Julian. "Consciousness and the Voices of the Mind." *Canadian Psychology / Psychologie canadienne*, Vol. 27, No. 2, April 1986, pp. 1–17.

Jentsch, Ernst. *On the Psychology of the Uncanny* [1906]. Translated by Roy Sellars. *Angelaki: Journal of the Theoretical Humanities*, Vol. 2, No. 1, 1996, pp. 7–16. Published online: 4 June 2008. https://doi.org/10.1080/09697259708571910.

Kayser, Wolfgang. *The Grotesque in Art and Literature*. Translated by Ulrich Weisstein. Indiana University Press, 1963.

Kermode, Frank. *The Sense of an Ending: Studies in the Theory of Fiction.* Oxford University Press, 1967.

Kövecses, Zoltán. *Metaphor: A Practical Introductio*n. Oxford University Press, 2002.

Kristeva, Julia. *Powers of Horror: An Essay on Abjection.* Translated by Leon S. Roudiez. Columbia University Press, 1982.

Lacan, Jacques. *Anxiety.* Edited by Jacques-Alain Miller. Translated by A. R. Price. Polity Press, 2016.

Laplanche Jean, Serge Leclaire, and Patrick Coleman. "The Unconscious: A Psychoanalytic Study." *Yale French Studies*: *French Freud: Structural Studies in Psychoanalysis*, No. 48, 1972, pp. 118–75.

Lemke J. L. "More Than Cool Reason: A Field Guide to Poetic Metaphor." Review of *More Than Cool Reason: A Field Guide to Poetic Metaphor*, by George Lakoff and Mark Turner. *Linguistics and Education*, Vol. 4, 1992, pp. 247–53.

Levin, Samuel R. *The Semantics of Metaphor.* Johns Hopkins University Press, 2019.

Lodge, David. *Language of Fiction: Essays in Criticism and Verbal Analysis of the English Novel.* Columbia University Press, 1966.

Luther, Martin. *Luther's Works*, vol. 1. Lectures on Genesis 1–5, 1:2 [W, XLII 12, 13]. Edited by Jaroslav Pelikan. Concordia, 1958.

MacLeish, Archibald. "Ars Poetica." *Collected Poems 1917–1982.* Houghton Mifflin, 1985, pp. 106–7.

Masschelein, Anneleen. *The Unconcept: The Freudian Uncanny in Late-Twentieth-Century Theory.* State University of New York Press, 2011.

Matz, Robert. *Defending Literature in Early Modern England: Renaissance Literary Theory in Social Context*. Cambridge University Press, 2000.

Melaney, William. "Rancière's Proust: A Rebirth of Aesthetics," *Res Cogitans*, Vol. 13, No. 1, 2018, pp. 52–62.

Milton, John. *Areopagitica. The John Milton Reading Room*: *The Complete Poetry and Selected Prose of John Milton, with Introductions, Research Guides, and Hyperlinked Annotations.* Thomas H. Luxon, General Editor. © Trustees of Dartmouth College, 1997–2020. https://www.dartmouth.edu/~milton/reading_room/areopagitica/text.html.

Mitsi, Efterpi. "The 'popular philosopher': Plato, Poetry, and Food in Tudor Aesthetics." *Early Modern Literary Studies*, Vol. 9, No. 2, September 2003, pp. 1–23.

Morlock, Forbes. "Doubly Uncanny: An Introduction to 'On the Psychology of the Uncanny.'" *Angelaki: Journal of the Theoretical Humanities*, Vol. 2, No. 1, 1997, pp. 17–21. DOI: 10.1080/09697259708571911.

Morris, Charles Morris. *Signs, Language and Behavior.* Prentice-Hall, 1946.

Newman, John Henry. *The Idea of a University.* Edited by Martin J. Svaglic. Holt Rinehart, Winston, 1964.

Nietzsche, Friedrich. *The Portable Nietzsche*. Edited and translated by Walter Kaufmann. Viking, 1954.

Nordquist, Richard. "The Power and Pleasure of Metaphor." *ThoughtCo*, February 16, 2021. thoughtco.com/power-and-pleasure-of-metaphor-1689249

Nowottny, Winifred. *The Language Poets Use.* Athlone Press, 1975.

Ortega y Gasset, José. *The Dehumanization of Art; And Other Essays on Art, Culture, and Literature*. Princeton University Press, 1968.

Ortony, Andrew. "Why Metaphors Are Necessary and Not Just Nice." *Educational Theory*, Vol. 25, 1975, pp. 45–53.

Otto, Rudolf. *The Idea of the Holy: An Inquiry into the Non-Rational Factor in the Idea of the Divine and Its Relation to the Rational*, 2nd edition. Translated by John W. Harvey. Oxford University Press, 1950. First published as *Das Heilige* in 1917.

Percy, Walker. "Metaphor as Mistake." *The Sewanee Review*, Vol. 66, No. 1, Winter 1958, pp. 79–99.

Pierson, David Lawrence. *Narratives of Newark (in New Jersey) from the Days of Its Founding.* Pierson Publishing Co., 1917.

Plato. *Republic*. Translated by C. D. C. Reeve. Hackett, 2004.

Platt, Peter G. "'The Meruailouse [sic] Site': Shakespeare, Venice, and Paradoxical Stages." *Renaissance Quarterly*, Vol. 54, No. 1, Spring 2001. Gale Literature Resource Center. link.gale.com/apps/doc/A74523890/LitRC?u=cornell&sid=bookmark-LitRC&xid=a0034c28. n. pag., paragraph 12.

Punter, David. *Metaphor.* Routledge, 2007.

Puttenham, George. *Arte of English Poesie*. https://www.gutenberg.org/cache/epub/16420/pg16420.html, p. 189.

Rancière, Jacques. *Mute Speech.* Translated by James Swenson. Columbia University Press, 2011.

Richards, I. A. *The Philosophy of Rhetoric.* Oxford University Press, 1936.

Ricoeur, Paul. *The Rule of Metaphor: Multidisciplinary Studies of the Creation of Meaning in Language*. Translated by Robert Czerny, with Kathleen McLaughlin and John Costello, SJ. University of Toronto Press, 1977.

Ross, John Robert. *Constraints on Variables in Syntax.* Ph.D. Thesis. MIT, Dept. of Modern Languages and Linguistics, 1967.

Royle, Nicholas. *The Uncanny.* Routledge, 2003.

Sapir, J. David. "The Anatomy of Metaphor." *The Social Use of Metaphor: Essays on the Anthropology of Rhetoric.* Edited by J. David Sapir and J. Christopher Crocker. University of Pennsylvania Press, 1977, pp. 3–32.

Savage, Robert. "Introduction." Hans Blumenberg, *Paradigms for a Metaphorology.* Translated from the German with an afterword by Robert Savage. Cornell University Press and Cornell University Library, 2010, pp. 1–5.

Schelling, F. W. J. von, *Philosophie der Mythologie.* Edited by K. F. A. Schelling. *Sämtliche Werke* 2.2. G. Cotta, 1857.

Sparshott, F. E., "'As,' or the Limits of Metaphor." *New Literary History*, Vol. 6, No. 1, Autumn 1974, pp. 75–94.

Stanford, W. Bedell. *Greek Metaphor: Studies in Theory and Practice*. Oxford University Press, 1936.

Steiner, George. *Martin Heidegger*. University of Chicago Press, 1991.

Stevens, Wallace. *Opus Posthumous*. Edited by Milton J. Bates. Alfred Knopf, 1989.

Swift, Jonathan. *A Tale of a Tub*, … Edited by A. C. Guthkelch and D. Nichol Smith. Clarendon Press, 1920.

Todorov, Tzvetan. "Synecdoques." *Communications*, No. 16, 1970, pp. 26–35.

Turbayne, Colin. *The Myth of Metaphor*. Yale University Press, 1962.

Turner, V[ictor]. W. *Chihamba the White Spirit: A Ritual Drama of the Ndembu*. Published on behalf of The Rhodes-Livingstone Institute by Manchester University Press, 1962.

Vaihinger, Hans. *The Philosophy of "As If,"* 2nd edition. Translated by C. K. Ogden. Routledge & Kegan Paul, 1935.

Valéry, Paul. "Philosophy of the Dance." *What Is Dance? Readings in Theory and Criticism*. Translated by Ralph Manheim. Edited by Roger Copeland and Marshall Cohen. Oxford University Press, 1983.

Watt, Ian. *The Rise of the Novel: Studies in Defoe, Richardson, and Fielding*. Chatto & Windus, 1957.

Wikipedia, s.v. "Darmok." https://en.wikipedia.org/wiki/Darmok.

Wimsatt, William K., Jr., and Cleanth Brooks. *Literary Criticism: A Short History*. Alfred A. Knopf, 1957.

Windsor, Mark. "Freud on the Uncanny: A Tale of Two Theories." *Philosophy and Literature*, Vol. 44, No. 1, April 2020, pp. 35–51.

Withy, Katherine. *Heidegger on Being Uncanny*. Harvard University Press, 2015.

Wittgenstein, Ludwig. *Philosophische Untersuchungen/Philosophical Investigations*. Translated by G. E. M. Anscombe, P. M. S. Hacker, and Joachim Schulte, revised 4th edition by P. M. S. Hacker and Joachim Schulte. This fourth edition first published 2009 © 2009 Blackwell Publishing Ltd.

Woolf, Virginia. *To the Lighthouse*. Wordsworth Editions, 1994.

Zanker, Andreas T. *Greek and Latin Expressions of Meaning: The Classical Origins of a Modern Metaphor*. New edition [online]. C.H. Beck, 2016. http://books.openedition.org/chbeck/1609. DOI: https://doi.org/10.4000/books.chbeck.1609.

Zill, Rüdiger. "Der Fallensteller: Hans Blumenberg als Historiograph der Wahrheit." *Zeitschrift für Ideengeschichte*, Vol. 1, No. 3, 2007, pp. 21–38.

Žižek, Slavoj (ed.). *Everything You Always Wanted to Know about Lacan (But Were Afraid to Ask Hitchcock)*. Verso, 1992.

INDEX

abjection 58
Abrams, M. H. 2, 95–7
abstraction 5, 10, 25
Ambrose, Saint 31, 33
animism 64–5
Anker, Elizabeth S. 85
Aristotle 1, 12, 66, 84, 95
Auden, W. H. 8
Auerbach, Erich 27–9, 35–7
Augustine of Hippo, Saint 29–30, 32–4, 40–1, 92

back-formation (linguistic) 46
Bacon, Francis 43
Barany, Michael 18–19
Barthes, Roland 58
Beardsley, Monroe 47, 59
beauty 10, 33, 89–92
Berggren, Douglas 38–40
Berryman, John 71
bias 8–9
Black, Max 2, 14, 24–5, 37, 43, 56, 84, 96
Blackmur, R. P. 14, 45
Blackwell, Mark 48
Blake, William 67
Blumenberg, Hans 25, 35–6, 40, 53, 62, 68
Bogel, Fredric V. 38, 71, 72
Borch-Jacobsen, Mikkel 89
Boswell, James 65
Bresnick, Adam 73–4
Breton, André 16–17
Brooke-Rose, Christine 12–13
Brooks, Cleanth 84
Browne, Sir Thomas 83, 86
Burke, Edmund 4–6
Burke, Kenneth 1, 13–14, 55
Butler, Bishop Joseph 7, 15, 32–3, 60, 87–8

Cassirer, Ernst 43–4, 57, 67
Christianity 26–34, 51, 85–7
Cicero 32
circumstance 5
Coleridge, Samuel Taylor 61
Colie, Rosalie L. 85
container and contained 27, 29–31
convincing 63
crazing 92
Crocker, J. Christopher 3
Culler, Jonathan 16, 18, 81–2
culture and society 39, 58–9; novelty in 66–7; paradox and 85; ritual 80–2; shock/violence 72, 77; sociocultural uncanny 61–5, 79; theories of metaphor 2–3
Cureton, Richard D. 23

"Darmok" *see Star Trek*
Davidson, Donald 96
de Man, Paul 4, 43

death 49–51, 53, 58, 70–2, 77, 85–6, 92
Derrida, Jacques 1, 68–9, 81
dialectic 60, 85
Dickinson, Emily 8–9, 93
Diderot, Denis 48, 52
disorder 80–4
dogma 26
Donoghue, Dennis 2, 14, 16, 28–9, 32, 54–5
doubleness 28–9, 35–6, 48, 50, 58, 69–72, 74–5
Douglas, Mary 80–2, 85, 88–9

education 19–21
Eliot, T. S. 76, 85
Empson, William 17–18, 21, 58
Engh, Line Cecilie 29
epitaphs 50
erasure 69
etymology 36–7, 69
Everett, Percival 2
Exodus 33–4

Ferber, Michael 25
fictionality 8, 40, 42–7, 49, 51–3
Fielding, Henry 38–41, 61
figural interpretation 27–9, 35–6
Fitzgerald, F. Scott 11, 13, 16
Florio, John 84
Freud, Sigmund 10, 20, 45, 58–62, 64–5, 70–4, 76–9, 81
Fried, Debra 50
Frost, Robert 1, 7–8, 33
Frye, Northrop 1, 23, 28, 45

Gallie, W. B. 43
Gass, William 68
Girard, René 62, 72, 80
Goodman, Nelson 9, 22–3, 35–6
Gosson, Stephen 42
Griffith, Susan Blackburn 29–32, 34
grotesque 70

Hamlet 8, 65
Heidegger, Martin 36
Hertz, Neil 52, 72
Hester, Marcus B. 2, 4, 13
Hills, David 35–6
Hopkins, Gerard Manley 44, 92
Horace 39, 45
Hughes, Ted 48, 52
Husserl, Edmund 35

indirectness *see* obliquity
it-narratives 47–8, 52

Jakobson, Roman K. 12
James, William 25
Jameson, Fredric 82
Jarrell, Randall 49, 52
Jaynes, Julian 61, 66–7
Jentsch, Ernst 14, 20, 58, 61, 73–4, 81
Johnson, Mark 3
Johnson, Samuel 38, 65
Johnstone, Charles 48

Kayser, Wolfgang 70
Kermode, Frank 19, 40
Kierkegaard, Søren 51
Kövecses, Zoltán 3
Kristeva, Julia 58

Lacan, Jacques 41, 58–9, 70–1
Lakoff, George 3
Laplanche, Jean 25
Lele people 80–1
Levin, Samuel R. 23
lightning 8–9, 93
Locke, John 4, 39
Lodge, David 45–6
Luther, Martin 34

MacLeish, Archibald 84
Malamud, Bernard 2, 65
Marx, Karl 51
Masschelein, Anneleen 78
Melaney, William 58
metaphier and metaphrand *see* Jaynes, Julian
metaphor: as assertion of identity 6–7, 10–13; as category mistake 16, 24; and Christianity 26–34, 51, 85–7, *see also* typology; as discovery or creation 13–14, 43–4, 66–7; as double synecdoche 7; as foundational 24–6; and indirectness 7–9; and mathematics 18–19; and mistake 14, 44–5, 57; modes of analysis 2–6; as narrative of education 19–21; and ontology 12–13, 26, 44–5, 54–5; and prophecy 54–5; readerly processing of 15–18; and redefinition 11–13, 15–16, 24, 41, 67–8; and "seeing as" 13, 24, 55–6; and simile 12–13, 16, 66, 75, 95–6; and temporality 18–19; tenor and vehicle of 6–7; theories of 2–4, 6–7, 24–6, 95–7; truth and falsity of 7–10, 13–14, 16–26, 40–9, 51–3, 59–60; and the uncanny 58–65, 67–74, 76–87; views of 1–2, 10
metaphor and paradox 41, 59–60, 83–5, 87, 91–3

metaphor and religion 26–34, 51, 83, 85–7
metaphor and wonder 83–4, 86–7
Milton, John 19, 87, 90–2
Möbius strip 70–1, 73
Morris, Charles 7

Newman, John Henry 3–4
Nietzsche, Friedrich 81–2
noun-forms 46
Nowottny, Winifred 44

obliquity 7–9, 23, 33, 74, 93
Ortega y Gasset, José 2
Ortony, Andrew 12–13
Otto, Rudolf 86
Ovid 28
oxymoron 59–60

paradox 41, 59–60, 83–5, 87, 91–3
parapraxes 45, 78–9
Pascal, Blaise 7, 68–9
Patrizi, Francesco 84
Percy, Walker 14, 44–5, 57–8
pharmakon 81, 89
Plato (*Republic*) 18–22, 42; and illusion vs. reality 20–2
Platt, Peter G. 84–5
Plotinus 89–92
poems, as metaphors: Ch. 6 (*passim*)
Pope, Alexander 63, 74
Potter, Dennis 66
properness 63
psychoanalysis *see* uncanny
Punter, David 60
purity and impurity 80, 83, 87–93; in Dickinson 93; in Hopkins (Gerard Manley) 92; in Milton 90–2; in Plotinus 89–91; in Yeats 91, *see also* Douglas, Mary
Puttenham, George 84

Raine, Craig 47, 52
Rancière, Jacques 83–4
Rank, Otto 71, 83
rationality and the non-rational 5, 83–7
Real (Lacanian) 58, 70
realism (genre) 23, 45
reality 14, 20–4, 43–5, 64, 67, 81–2
reference (and referentiality) 43, 45–6
religion 26–34, 51, 83, 85–7
Renaissance 42, 45, 84
repression 14, 59, 62–4, 68, 72–3, 76–9, 81
reservoir, cultural 59, 62–4, 67, 79
resistance, readerly 16–18, 21–2, 35, 58, 87
revolutions 4–5
Richards, I. A. 1–2, 6, 37, 61, 95–6
Ricoeur, Paul 12, 24, 56, 59–60, 65
ritual 80–1, 84–5
Royle, Nicholas 63
Ryle, Gilbert 24

Sapir, J. David 3, 35
Savage, Robert 36, 62
scaffolding, metaphor as 31, 34
Schelling, F. W. J. von 62, 68, 77
self and other 54, 56–8; ego 63–4, 66, 71, 73–5
Shakespeare, William 8, 11, 13, 16, 42, 65
Shelley, Percy 7, 39, 67–8
shock 21, 23, 58, 73, 76–7, 79
Sidney, Philip 43
society *see* culture and society
Sontag, Susan 3
Stanford, W. Bedell 38
Star Trek 74–5
Steiner, George 36
stereoscopic vision 38–9, 74
Stern, Gustav 17
Stevens, Wallace 22, 24–5, 54
Surrealism 16–17
Swift, Jonathan 33, 89
synecdoche, double 7

Tannen, Deborah 3
tenor and vehicle 6–7, 15–19, 95–6; biblical interpretation 27, 29, 31–3; doubling 70–1, 73–6; identity of 10, 12; persistence of the tenor 35–41; self and other 54, 56–7; truth and falsity 22–3, 53; uncanny 58–9, 61, 63–8, 81
Tertullian 30–1, 86
Todorov, Tzvetan 7, 96
Trudeau, Garry 17
Turbayne, Colin 16, 24
Turner, Mark 3
Turner, Victor 84
typology 27–9, 37

uncanny 7, 14, 20, 41, 45, 58–87; doubling 69–75; in paradox and religion 83–7; psychoanalytic and sociocultural 61–5, 76–82; ritual and 80–2

Vaihinger, Hans 47
Valéry, Paul 1
verb-forms 46

Watt, Ian 45
Wimsatt, W. K. 56, 89–90
windlass 8
Windsor, Mark 64
Withy, Katherine 45, 69–70, 73–4, 78–9, 81, 85
Wittgenstein, Ludwig 13, 24, 48, 55
wonder 83–4, 86–7
Woolf, Virginia 33, 87
wrapping 29–34, 56
Wright, Steven 12

Yeats, W. B. 67, 91

Zill, Rüdiger 62
Žižek, Slavoj 70–1, 73